Meniere's Disease

Edited by Fayez Bahmad Jr.

Published in London, United Kingdom

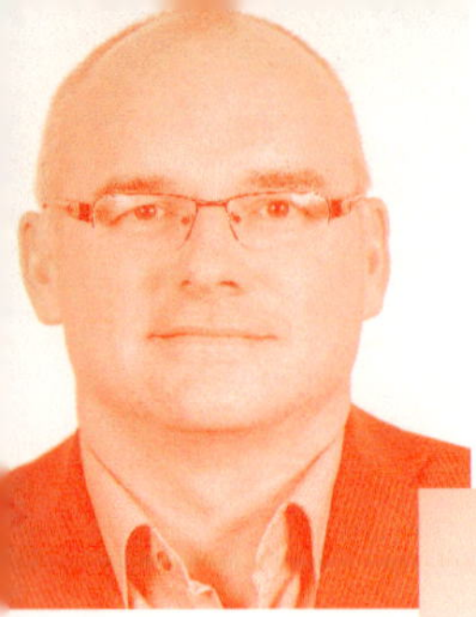
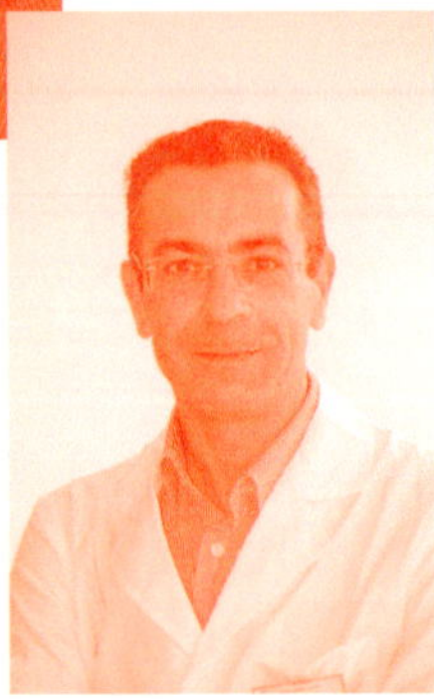
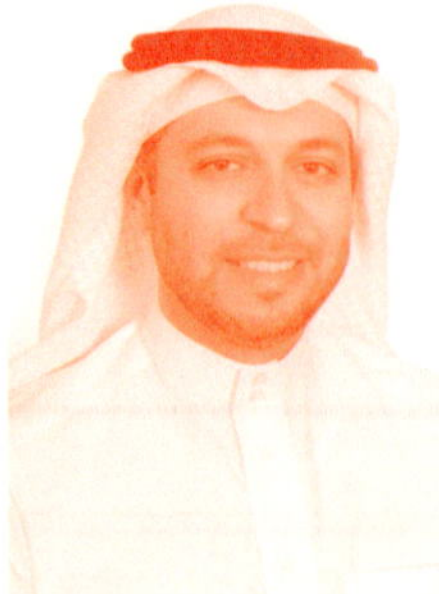
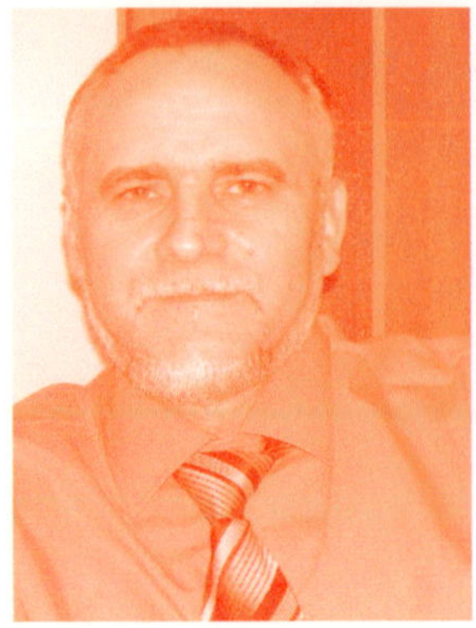
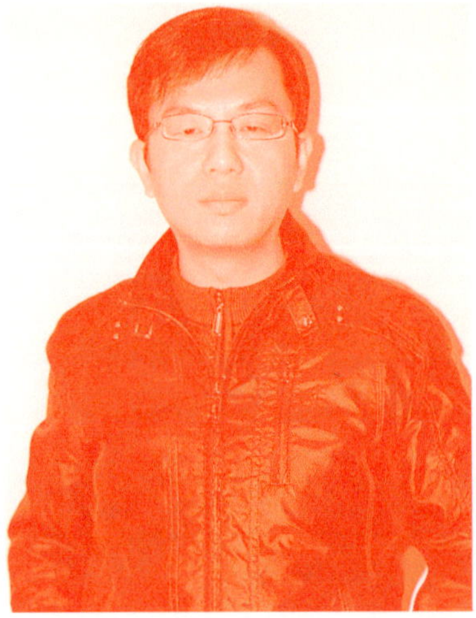
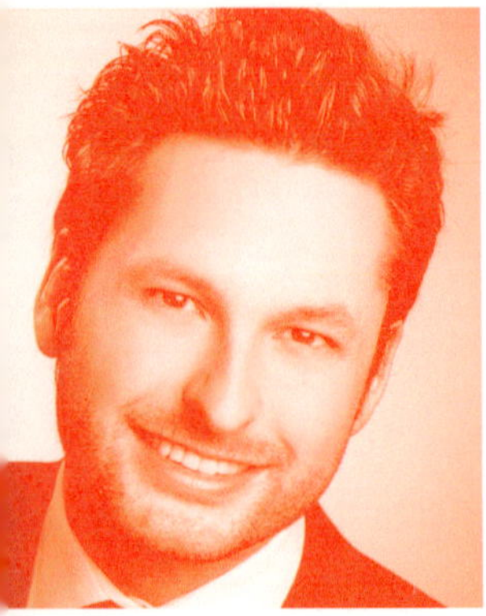
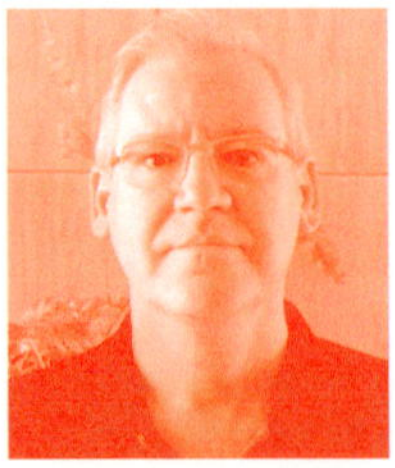

IntechOpen

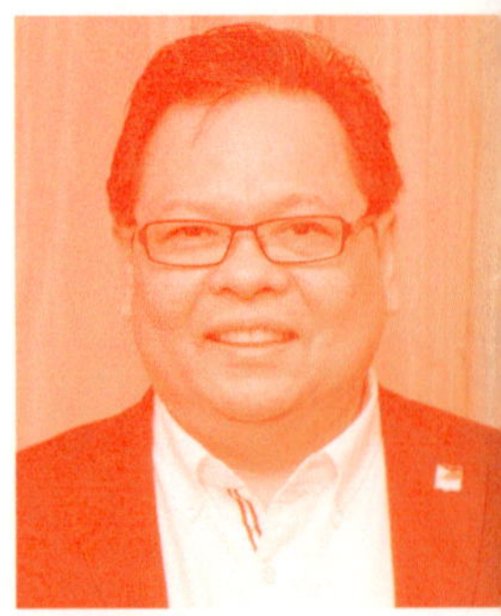
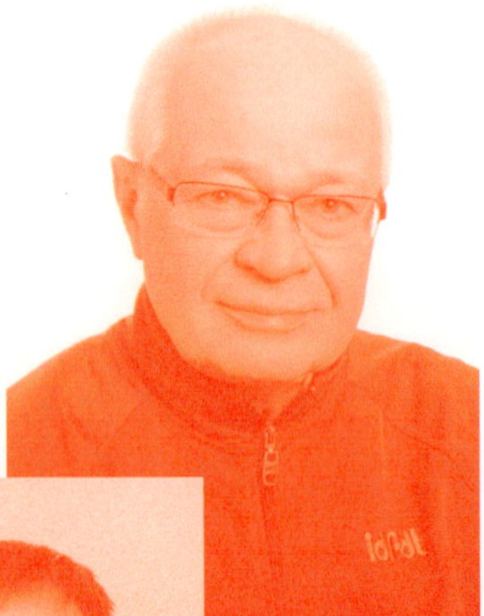
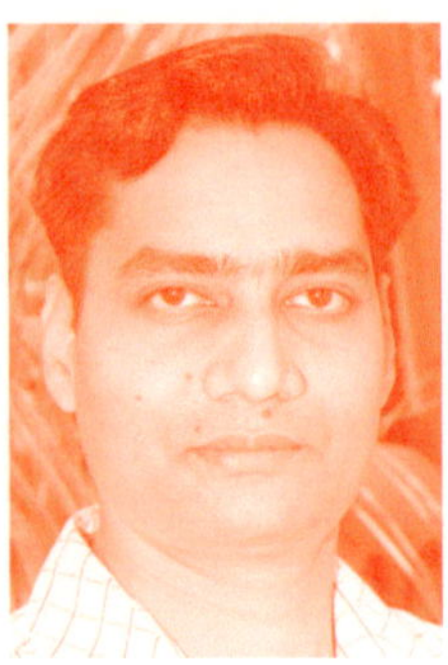
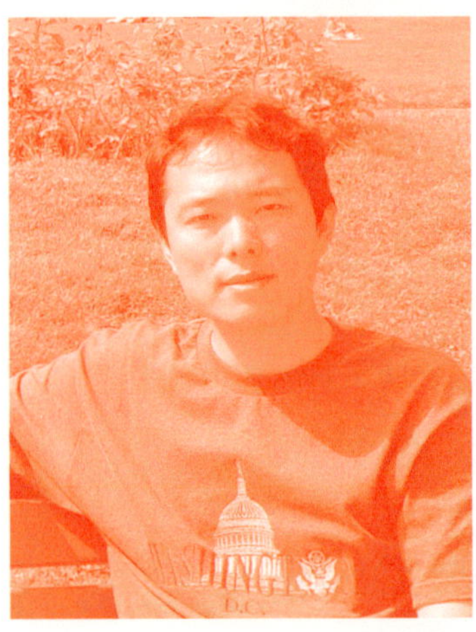
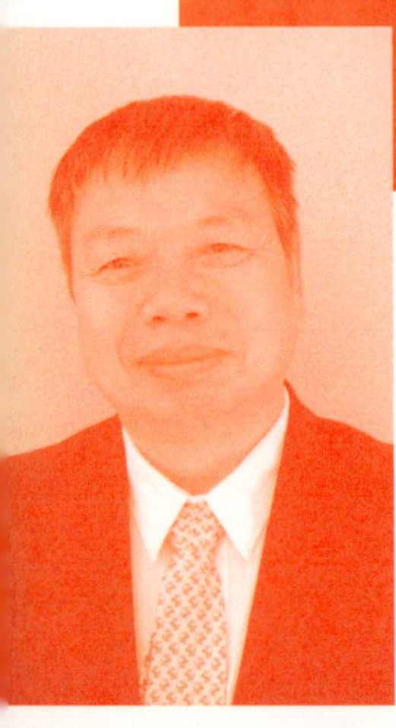
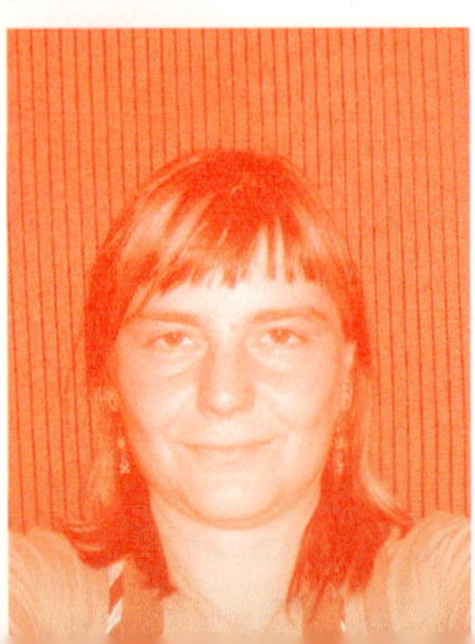

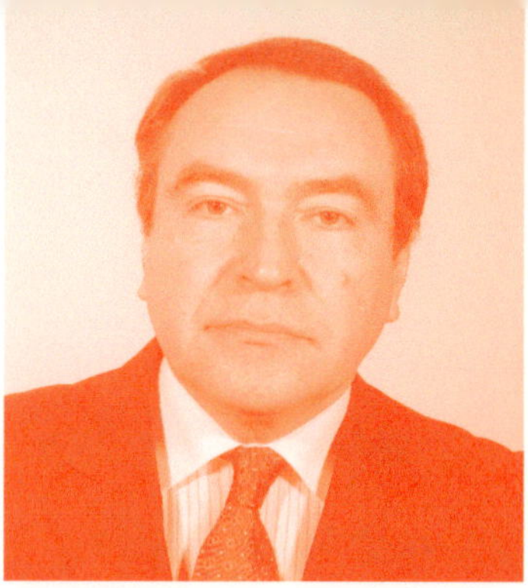
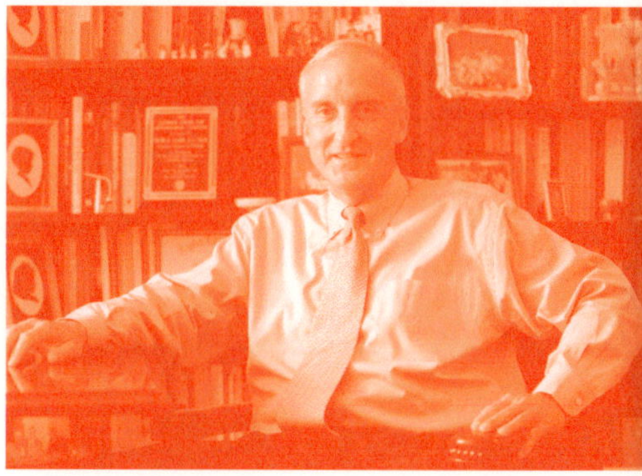
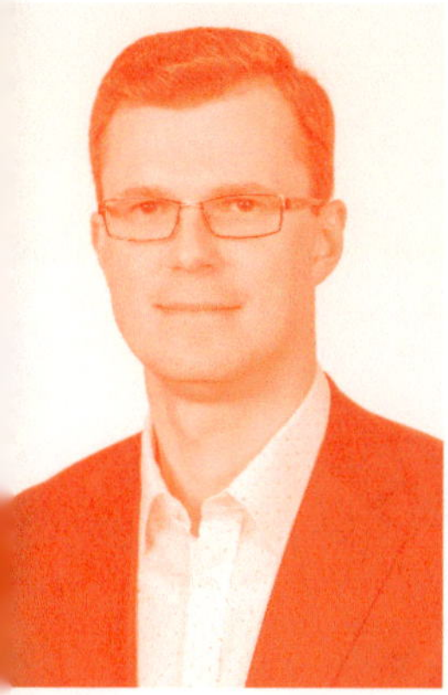
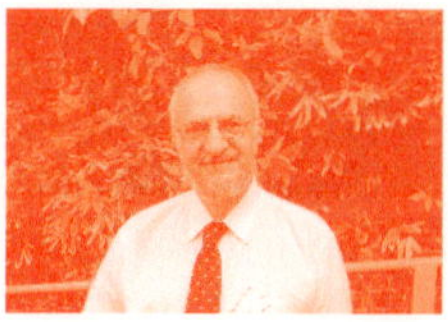
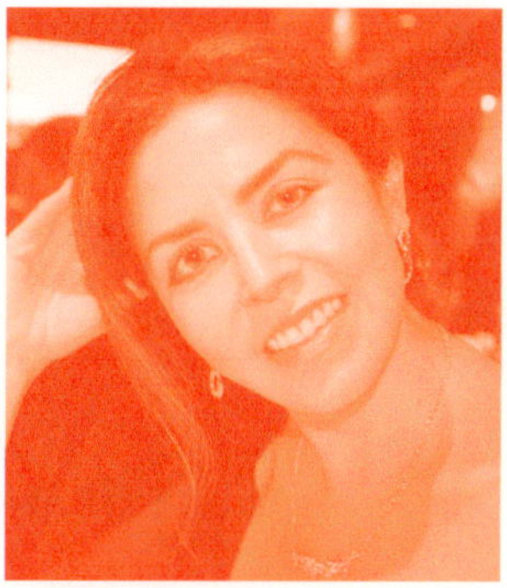

Supporting open minds since 2005

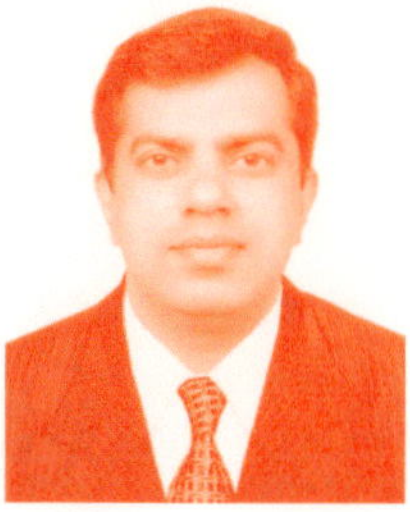
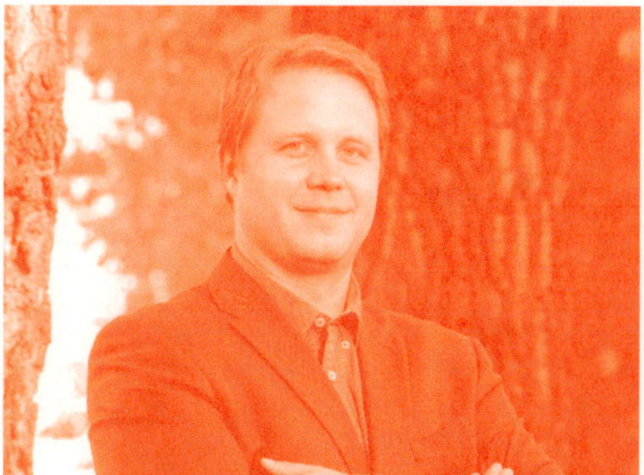
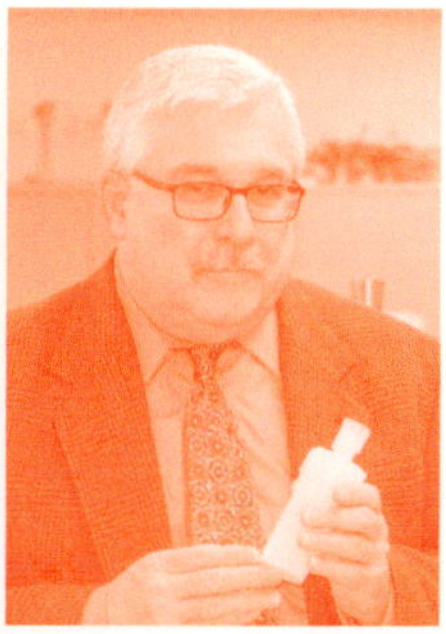
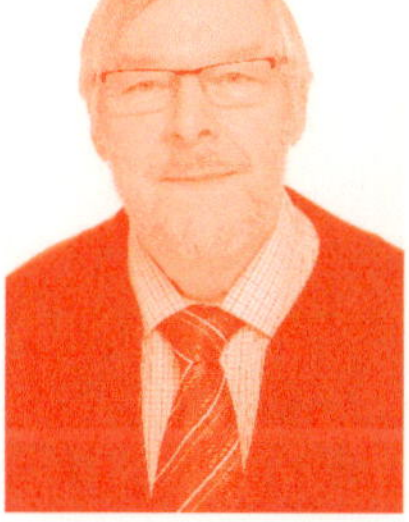
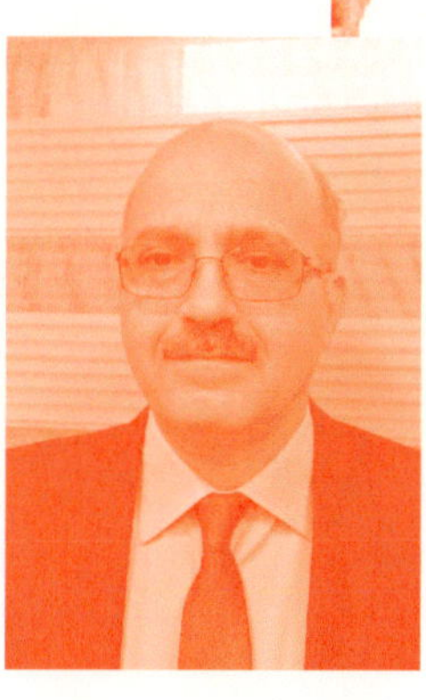
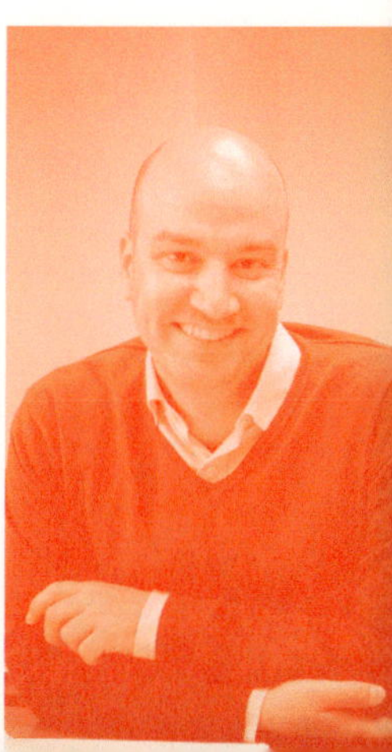
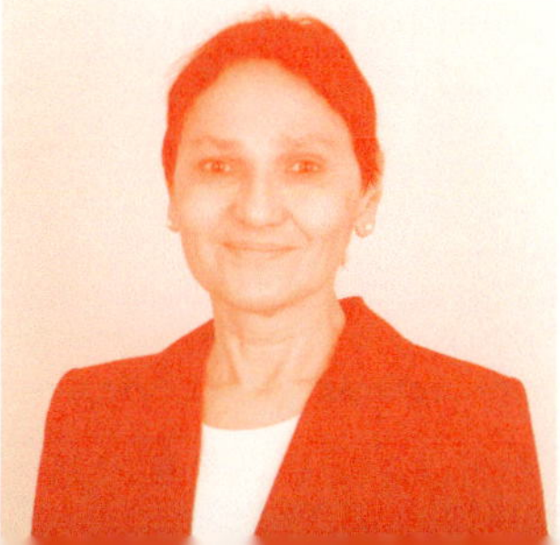

Meniere's Disease
http://dx.doi.org/10.5772/intechopen.77710
Edited by Fayez Bahmad Jr.

Contributors
Maria Stella Arantes Do Amaral, Henrique Furlan Pauna, Ana Cláudia M.B. Reis, Miguel Hyppolito, Mehmet Yilmaz, Yetkin Zeki Yilmaz, Begüm Bahar Yilmaz, Aysegul Batioglu-Karaaltin, Carlos Augusto C. P. Oliveira, Hongzhe Li, Yongchuan Chai, Paula Lopes, Ricardo Bento, Fayez Bahmad

First published in London, United Kingdom, 2020 by IntechOpen
IntechOpen is the global imprint of INTECHOPEN LIMITED, registered in England and Wales, registration number: 11086078, 7th floor, 10 Lower Thames Street, London, EC3R 6AF, United Kingdom
Printed in Croatia

British Library Cataloguing-in-Publication Data
A catalogue record for this book is available from the British Library

Additional hard and PDF copies can be obtained from orders@intechopen.com

Meniere's Disease
Edited by Fayez Bahmad Jr.
p. cm.
Print ISBN 978-1-78923-939-3
Online ISBN 978-1-78923-940-9
eBook (PDF) ISBN 978-1-83880-551-7

For EU product safety concerns:
IN TECH d.o.o., Prolaz Marije Krucifikse Kozulić 3, 51000 Rijeka, Croatia, info@intechopen.com or visit our website at intechopen.com.

Meet the editor

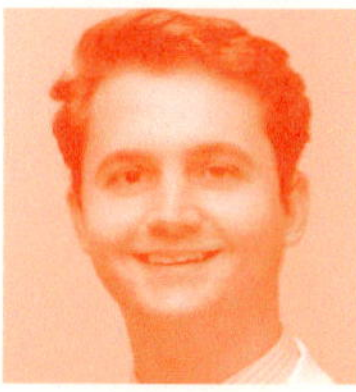

Professor Fayez Bahmad Jr. is a doctor of medicine and specialist in otology and neurotology. He lives in Brasilia (the Brazilian capital). He did an ENT residency program at the University of Brasilia Hospital in otolaryngology between 2002 and 2005, and received his PhD from the University of Brasilia—Medical School under the orientation of Professor Carlos A. Oliveira, MD, PhD. Professor Oliveira established an otopathology laboratory in his department, which is one of the most well-respected research groups in otology in Brazil and South America. Professor Bahmad received a Fellowship in Otology and Neurotology from the Massachusetts Eye and Ear Infirmary, Harvard Medical School, and a Fellowship in Human Genetics from the Seidman Laboratory, Department of Genetics, Harvard Medical School, where he was engaged in research projects under the mentorship of Professor Saumil N. Merchant MD, PhD, and Professor Jonathan Seidman MD, two of the foremost researchers in otology, otopathology, and hearing pathogenetics. In 2019 he became Professor Livre-docente of Ophthalmology and Otorhinolaryngology, Department of the University of Sao Paulo, Sao Paulo, Brazil. He has experience in medicine, focusing on otological surgery, acting in the following subjects: hearing loss and tinnitus. He is the Director of the Brasiliense Institute of Otolaryngology, editor in chief of *The International Tinnitus Journal*, and a professor at the Health Science Faculty at the University of Brasilia, Brazil.

Contents

Preface

Ménière's disease is an alteration of the inner ear characterized by two groups of symptoms: vestibular symptoms and auditory symptoms. Classical symptoms such as fluctuating hearing loss, tinnitus, atrial fullness, and concomitant dizziness greatly aid the otorhinolaryngologist to diagnose carriers of the disease. But in many patients, their presentation may be different.

In this book we will adopt the term Ménière's disease to follow the prevailing trend among most research groups and discuss the main topics and current and past ideas about the etiopathogenesis, diagnosis, and treatment of Ménière's disease and Ménière's disease associated with migraine.

It is likely that there are genotypic—racial as well as phenotypic—environmental factors that influence the prevalence difference between countries. One of the major problems in this respect is that the initial presentation of the disease is often the cochlear form, which is not clinically recognized, and is again attributed to another specific cause or is presumed to be simply due to aging. Even after the vestibular component becomes obvious, long periods of remission may mask the complete final image of the syndrome with episodic vertigo, fluctuating autistic loss, tinnitus, and aural fullness. Therefore, generally, in clinical practice, only moderate to severe cases have been tabulated in the estimates so far.

Some of the epidemiologically published studies to date have tended to blend different epidemiological concepts. The direction of these studies is mainly retrospective (the themes are identified after a result or illness), and they actually measure only prevalence (existing events or the number of cases of a disease at a given moment divided by the population at risk). Only prospective studies (subjects are identified before a result or illness, and future events are counted) would have the power to adequately measure this incidence. Although more reflective of real life than an artificial experiment, retrospective observational studies are susceptible to bias.

The multiplicity of diagnostic criteria is another problem that makes it difficult to establish the true incidence of Ménière's disease in the general population. In 1972 the Committee on Hearing and Equilibrium of the American Academy of Otorhinolaryngology proposed a specific definition of the disease and guidelines for the evaluation of Ménière's disease in communicating treatment results. In 1985, it was considered that the definition of Ménière's disease needed to be restricted to cases with a complete set of classic signs and symptoms. The 1995 criteria were intended to simplify the definition of Ménière's disease and allow greater flexibility, making it usable in a wide range of studies and classifications. A minimum set of signs and symptoms must be noted in such a way that the degree of certainty of the diagnosis can be established.

Currently, there is no universally accepted theory about the pathophysiology of this disease. Through histopathological studies, it is presumed that endolymphatic hydrops is the most descriptive pathological characteristic of Ménière's disease.

The pathophysiology of the symptoms is still disputed: ruptures of membranes, increased pressure and mechanical displacement of the peripheral organs as saccule by endolymph accumulation, viral infections, and autoimmune disease in addition to several other theories that have already been reported. It can be seen that in this scheme, currently accepted endolymphatic hydrops is no longer a central etiology but rather one of the manifestations of the syndrome. And the exact mechanism of the etiopathogenesis of the syndrome remains unknown. It is believed that multifactorial inheritance is the best response, in which the necessary conditions are met to lead to malabsorption of the endolymph and, subsequently, to dropsy. Clinical and laboratory evidence supports this concept.

Fayez Bahmad Jr.
University of Brasilia,
Brasilia, DF, Brazil

Ophthalmology and Otolaryngology Faculty,
University of São Paulo,
São Paulo, SP, Brazil

Section 1

Introduction

Chapter 1

Introductory Chapter: Ménière's Disease (MD)

Fayez Bahmad Jr

1. Introduction

Ménière's disease (MD) is probably a multifactorial disorder where the genetics and environmental factors determine the onset of the disease. This disease have been related to the accumulation of endolymph in the cochlear duct and the vestibular organs in histopathological studies, although endolymphatic hydrops (EH) per se does not explain all clinical features, including the progression of hearing loss or the frequency of attacks of vertigo [1–4].

Dizziness and vertigo are frequent symptoms in the otolaryngologist's practice, and all efforts towards the better comprehension of this system and its pathology are of fundamental importance [1, 2].

Currently, there is no universally accepted theory about the pathophysiology of the disease. Through histopathological studies, it is assumed that endolymphatic hydrops is the most descriptive pathological feature of Ménière's disease. The pathophysiology of symptoms is still widely disputed: membrane ruptures, increased pressure, and mechanical displacement of peripheral organs such as endolymph accumulation, viral infections, autoimmune disease, and several other theories that have been reported [1–3].

Great advances have been made in neuro-otology, and increasing knowledge in the field of molecular biology, genetics, and neurosciences has substantially modified the approach of the patient with balance complaints. This book studies the most interesting and controversial of these vestibular diseases, the Ménière's disease.

The Classification Committee for the International Classification of Vestibular Disorders (ICVD) nominated by the Bárány Society, 2009, standardized the nomenclature of vestibular symptoms (SV) in four groups. One of the most important is the episodic vestibular syndrome: crises of vestibular symptoms interspersed with asymptomatic periods, such as Ménière's syndrome and vestibular migraine [1, 2–6].

Ménière's disease is an inner ear alteration characterized by two groups of symptoms: vestibular and auditory symptoms. In many patients, their presentation may be unusual or different than the classical symptoms such as tinnitus, fluctuating hearing loss, aural fullness, and concomitant dizziness [1, 2].

The history of the disease may be progressive or nonprogressive, and, in addition to the typical clinical presentation of Ménière's disease, two variants of the disease were identified:

1. cochlear Ménière's disease—hearing is the predominant symptom; and

2. vestibular Ménière's disease—vestibular symptoms are predominant.

Other classifications used frequently are as follows:

1. Ménière's syndrome: known and well-established condition causing symptoms; and

2. Ménière's disease: idiopathic cause [1, 2].

Recent studies revealed that there are genotypic and phenotypic factors that influence the prevalence difference between countries [7].

In the majority of these patients, the initial presentation of the disease is often the cochlear form, which is harder to be clinically recognized and frequently is associated with another cause or is presumed to be simply due to aging.

Even after the vestibular component becomes obvious, long periods of remission may mask the complete final image of the syndrome with episodic vertigo, fluctuating autistic loss, tinnitus, and aural fullness. Therefore, generally in clinical practice, only moderate to severe cases are tabulated in the estimates so far.

A multifactorial inheritance is believed to be the best response, where the necessary conditions are met, leading to endolymph malabsorption and subsequently hydrops. Clinical and laboratory evidence supports this concept. Merchant et al. analyzed the temporal bone collection of the Massachusetts Eye and Ear Infirmary, Harvard Medical School, Boston, USA, with a clinical diagnosis of Ménière's syndrome (28 cases) or a histopathological diagnosis of hydrops (79 cases).

All 28 cases with classic symptoms of Ménière's syndrome had hydrops in at least one ear. However, the reverse is not true. There were 9 cases of idiopathic hydrops and 10 cases with secondary hydrops, in which the patients did not have the classic symptoms of Ménière's syndrome. Endolymph is mainly produced in the stria vascularis. Slowly, endolymph is absorbed into the endolymphatic duct and sac, a biologically active transport structure where absorption occurs mainly and also to a lesser extent secretion occurs. Evidence strongly suggests that longitudinal flow (slow process) and radial flow (fast) occur.

In this book we will adopt the term Ménière's disease to follow the prevailing trend among most research groups and discuss the main topics, current and past ideas about etiopathogenesis, diagnosis, and treatment of Ménière's disease associated with migraine.

Some of the epidemiologically published studies to date have tended to blend different epidemiological concepts. The direction of these studies is mainly retrospective (the themes are identified after a result or illness), and they actually measure only the prevalence (existing events or the number of cases of a disease at a given moment divided by the population at risk). Only prospective studies (subjects are identified before a result or illness, future events are counted) would have the power to adequately measure this incidence. Although more reflective to real life than an artificial experiment, retrospective observational studies are susceptible to bias.

2. Diagnostic failures

There are many classifications and proposed diagnostic criteria, and it makes difficult to establish the true incidence of Ménière's disease in the general population.

The 1995 and 2015 criteria simplified the definition of Ménière's disease and allowed to be usable in all global studies and so may be able to substitute and unify all the classifications [1, 2].

3. Etiopathogeny

Almost all the researchers and histopathological works in the past presumed that endolymphatic hydrops was the pathological characteristic of Ménière's disease. There are still many questions and polemic discussions about the pathophysiology of the symptoms: increased pressure and mechanical displacement of the peripheral organs such as saccule by endolymph accumulation, ruptures of membranes, viral infections, and autoimmune disease, in addition to several other theories that have already been reported.

Recent consensus accepted that endolymphatic hydrops is no longer a central etiology but rather as one of the manifestations of the syndrome.

4. Diagnostic

Classical Ménière's disease is an excellent example of a condition that can be diagnosed on clinical grounds and simple audiometric examinations.

When it is the classic or definite form, it is characterized by recurrent and spontaneous episodes of vertigo, fluctuating sensorineural hearing loss, tinnitus, and aural fullness. In this case the diagnosis is easy even for the most naive clinician [1, 2].

In 2015, the Hearing and Balance Committee of the American Academy of Otorhinolaryngology-Head and Neck Surgery (AAO-HNS), Bárány Society, and other entities set the parameters for the clinical diagnosis of Ménière's disease.

The classification includes two categories: defined Ménière's disease and probable Ménière's disease [2].

Defined Ménière's disease is based on clinical criteria and requires the observation of an episodic vertigo syndrome associated with low- to medium-frequency sensorineural hearing loss and fluctuating auditory symptoms (tinnitus in the ear and/or fullness) in the affected ear.

The duration of vertigo episodes is limited to a period of between 20 minutes and 12 hours. Probable Ménière's disease is a broader concept defined by episodic vestibular symptoms (vertigo or dizziness) associated with fluctuating aural symptoms that occur over a period of 20 minutes to 24 hours [1, 2].

The clinical evaluation then includes the following [8, 9]:

- detailed medical history that should include all previous vertigo events;
- laboratory tests to rule out differential diagnoses of the syndrome;
- imaging tests to aid diagnosis and rule out differential diagnoses of the syndrome; and
- cochlear and vestibular, audiological, and electrophysiological examinations.

The most appropriate exams to aid in diagnosis consist of:

- glycerol dehydration test;
- electrocochleography (ECochG); and
- PEMV or VEMP test.

5. Treatment

Different treatment options for Ménière's disease exist with substantial variability between countries. None of the treatment options cure the disease. As many treatments have a significant impact on the functioning of surrounding structures, one should start with noninvasive approaches with the fewest possible side effects and proceed to more invasive steps:

- conservative;
- diet;
- diuretics;
- labyrinth suppressors;
- invasive procedures;
- intratympanic gentamicin;
- endolymphatic sac decompression surgery;
- labyrinthectomy; and
- vestibular neurectomy.

Sodium restriction diet: Low-level evidence suggests that restricting the sodium intake may help to prevent Ménière's attacks.

Betahistine: Substantial disagreement in the medical community about the use of betahistine exists. A Cochrane review found low-level evidence to support the use of betahistine with substantial variability between studies. Medical therapy in many medical centers often starts with betahistine orally.

Intratympanic steroid injections may reduce the number of vertigo attacks in patients with Ménière's disease.

Intratympanic gentamycin injections: Gentamycin has strong ablative properties towards vestibular cells. The side effects are a sensorineural hearing loss because of a certain amount of toxicity towards cochlear cells.

Surgery with vestibular nerve section or labyrinthectomy: Nerve section is a therapeutic option in patients who failed the conservative treatment options and labyrinthectomy when surgical options failed. Labyrinthectomy leads to a complete hearing loss in the affected side.

Clinically, three situations arise in which drug treatment is very helpful:

6. Acute attack drugs

Aiming at sedating the vestibule-trunk axis is particularly useful in aborting acute attacks. These include cinnarizine, promethazine, and diazepam.

Prolonged use of drugs such as cinnarizine is not advisable due to the risk of extrapyramidal side effects from prolonged use, particularly in the elderly.

6.1 Maintenance treatment

Dietary salt restriction and the use of diuretics such as furosemide, amiloride, and hydrochlorothiazide are attempts to prevent endolymphatic hydrops. The basis for this is historical rather than scientific, as the data from the few controlled studies that exist are conflicting and the placebo effect is clinically significant.

Betahistine has been subject to some scientific scrutiny, and several controlled clinical studies have shown significant improvement in vertigo, hearing loss, and tinnitus in the short term. Betahistine, with or without a diuretic, is currently the preferred means of ensuring medical treatment.

Drugs such as cinnarizine, propranolol (particularly if the patient has a history of migraine), and corticosteroids are also used empirically by some doctors if the patient's symptoms are refractory to the above measures.

7. Ablative treatment

7.1 Intratympanic gentamicin

The toxic effects of aminoglycosides on the inner ear sensory neuroepithelium have been recognized for decades.

Chemical labyrinthectomy through intratympanic gentamicin (GIT) controls vertigo and has been helpful in mainly unilateral Ménière's disease when hearing is poor, but the vertigo presented by the patient is disabling.

The attending otologist should properly remind and advise the patient that from 3 days after the first application, fiber differentiation begins to occur and this usually leads to severe vestibular symptoms between 7 and 10 days after application. And it is a phenomenon expected by the chemical destruction of vestibular nerve afferents.

Several series have a vertigo control rate of about 90%, although a cochleotoxic effect is seen in 15–25% of cases. The future for intratympanic aminoglycosides in Ménière's disease is therefore very promising [10].

Protocol of use:

- Complete battery of vestibular tests before therapy
- Initial reference (VENG before GIT)
- Provide for college entrance compensation
- Intratympanic gentamicin (40 mg/ml)
- Weekly intervals (up to three to four applications)
- Repeat audiometry weekly
- Repeat the VENG at the end of the sessions
- Topical anesthesia
- Patient rests for 1 hour after application

7.2 Surgical treatment

Whether as a result of medical treatment or as a consequence of the clinical course of Ménière's disease, about 90% of patients have a long period of remission.

This implies that 10% of patients continue to have clinically important episodes of vertigo, and surgical treatment should be considered for them.

The various surgical procedures advocated for Ménière's disease continue to raise considerable controversy among otolaryngologists. The decision to operate and the choice of procedure are often dictated by the understanding and experience of a particular technique and the surgeon's individual threshold for surgical intervention. Generally, surgical procedures for Ménière's disease are classified as destructive or nondestructive with regard to hearing [8–10].

7.3 Endolymphatic sac surgery

Endolymphatic sac surgery was first described in 1927 by Portmann, and no other aspect of Ménière's disease has elicited further debate or controversy. Just as the exact role of the endolymphatic sac in the development of hydrops is not yet known, the precise mechanism by which surgery works remains undefined. However, endolymphatic sac decompression surgery is still widely performed [10].

7.4 Vestibular nerve section

In the vestibular nerve section, no attempt is made to modify the underlying pathophysiology. The objective is to dissociate the offensive maze from the trunk, preserving the patient's hearing.

The procedure is uniformly effective, with vertigo control in 90–95% of patients according to some series. However, it is a surgery with considerable risks inherent in any posterior fossa neurosurgical procedure [10].

7.5 Surgical labyrinthectomy

Labyrinth extirpation is indicated in patients with severe symptoms who have virtually useless hearing. Disturbance of the inner ear thus invariably leads to permanent anacusis. However, the ear on the opposite side may have subclinical hydrops, and we should be naturally concerned that the progress of the disease in the patient's contralateral ear may aggravate and make it bilaterally deaf. This is probably the reason for the widespread choice of nondestructive inner ear procedures [10].

7.6 Cochlear implant

Over the past decade, the hearing rehabilitation of certain profoundly deaf people has been transformed by cochlear implants.

Patients with severe bilateral Ménière's disease and severe to profound bilateral sensorineural deafness will end up with an indication for hearing rehabilitation with cochlear implant. Surgeons with patients with symptoms whose disease is refractory to clinical treatment have several surgical options.

We should always start with the use of intratympanic aminoglycosides as the least aggressive option.

When intratympanic gentamicin does not work, there are three management strategies: proponents of endolymphatic sac surgery as the first surgical step, reserving revision surgery, or vestibular neurectomy for patients who continue to have vertigo.

Patients who have not yet achieved clinical improvement after the endolymphatic sac decompression operation, the otologist who has no experience or staff to subject the patient to vestibular neurectomy is faced with the option of performing surgical labyrinthectomy [10].

Author details

Fayez Bahmad Jr [1,2]

1 University of Brasilia, Brasilia, DF, Brazil

2 Ophthalmology and Otolaryngology Faculty, University of São Paulo (FMUSP), São Paulo, SP, Brazil

*Address all correspondence to: fayezbjr@gmail.com

References

[1] Members of the Committee on Hearing and Equilibrium. Committee on hearing and equilibrium, guidelines for the diagnosis and evaluation of therapy in Ménière's disease. Otolaryngology–Head and Neck Surgery. 1995;**113**:181-185

[2] Lopez-Escamez JA et al. Diagnostic criteria for Ménière's disease. Journal of Vestibular Research. 2015;**25**:1-7

[3] Oliveira CA, Bahmad F Jr, Sampaio AL. Ménière's Disease. In: Textbook of Vertigo - Diagnosis & Management. 1st ed. Vol. 01. New Delhi: Jaypee Brothers Medical Publishers; 2014. pp. 62-93

[4] Rauch SD, Merchant SN, Thedinger BA. Ménière's syndrome and endolymphatic hydrops: Double-blind temporal bone study. The Annals of Otology, Rhinology, and Laryngology. 1989;**98**:873-883

[5] Merchant SN, Adams JC, Nadol JB. Pathophysiology of Ménière' syndrome are symptoms caused by endolymphatic hydrops? Otology & Neurotology. 2005;**26**:74-81

[6] Agrawal Y, Minor LB. Ménière disease and other causes of episodic vertigo. In: Bronstein AM, editor. Vertigo and Imbalance. United Kingdom: Oxford; 2013. pp. 241-250

[7] Bahmad F Jr, DePalma SR, Merchant SN, Bezerra RL, Oliveira CA, Seidman CE, et al. Locus for familial migrainous vertigo disease maps to chromosome 5q35. The Annals of Otology, Rhinology, and Laryngology. 2009;**118**(9):670-676

[8] Cal R, Bahmad F Jr. Migraine associated with disfunção auditivo-vestibular auditory-vestibular dysfunction. BJORL. 2008;**74**(4):606-612

[9] Lamounier P, Gobbo DA, de Souza TSA, de Oliveira CACP, Bahmad F. Electrocochleography for Ménière's disease: Is it reliable? Brazilian Journal of Otorhinolaryngology. 2014;**80**:527-532

[10] Viana LM, Bahmad F Jr, Rauch SD. Intratympanic gentamicin as a treatment for drop attacks in patients with Ménière's disease. Laryngoscope. 2014;**124**(9):2151-2154

Section 2

Etiopathogenesis

Chapter 2

Menière's Disease: Etiopathogenesis

Carlos A. Oliveira

Abstract

This chapter will discuss idiopathic Menière's syndrome. That is to say—Menière's disease. We will start with a brief recall on the History of Menière's disease beginning with the description of the syndrome by Prosper Menière in 1861, the description of endolymphatic hydrops in temporal bone studies by Hallpike and Cairns in 1938 and by Yamakaua in the same year. Endolymphatic hydrops became a pathologic correlate for Menière's syndrome. Theories that considered endolymphatic hydrops as the cause of the syndrome will be discussed. More recent studies questioning the old theories and thinking of endolymphatic hydrops as an epiphenomenon in the course of the syndrome rather than the cause of the symptoms will be discussed. Temporal bone studies were the basis of these new theories too. Familial Menière's disease will be discussed and several families will be described in detail. Because the phenotype of siblings on each family studied was variable and migraine was present in many affected members of these families a spectrum was postulated going from migraine alone to full blown Menière's disease. Some siblings had what has been described recently as vertiginous migraine and a detailed description of this syndrome will be provided and the differences between this syndrome and Menière's disease will be made clear. About 20% of Menière's disease patients have a familial history. Sporadic Meniere's disease might have a genetic predisposition and other environmental and behavioral factors contribute for the surfacing of the disease (multifactorial etiology). Because migraine is a central phenomenon and the vertiginous episodes and auditory symptoms are peripheral a hypothesis is presented for the pathophysiology of Menière's disease. Recent research comparing vestibular migraine and Manière's disease reinforcing the concept of these syndromes representing a continuum process with similar etiology are discussed at the end.

Keywords: Menière's disease (MD), endolymphatic hydrops (EH), migraine, familial Menière's syndrome, continuum, vertiginous migraine (VM)

1. Introduction

This chapter will present the etiopathogenesis and pathophysiology of Menière's disease (MD). It is necessary therefore to make clear the definition of Menière's disease that will be considered here.

We consider Menière's disease the Menière's syndrome without a clear etiology. Because vertigo, tinnitus and hearing loss are present in most of the insults to the inner ear there are many known causes for these symptoms. However, there is the Menière's syndrome present in some patients without any definable etiology. This is Menière's disease and will be our subject in this chapter.

1.1 History of Menière's disease

Let us start with following the History of MD. In 1861 Prosper Menière suggested that vertigo, tinnitus and hearing loss were symptoms of vestibular organs injury rather than of brain apoplexy. This paper marked the starting point of a discussion that is now almost 180 years old [1].

In 1938 Hallpike and Cairns described in temporal bone histopathology study hydrops of the endolymphatic compartment in patients who had the Menière's symptoms during life. This was a material proof of the inner ear origin of the Menière's syndrome as stated by Menière in 1861 [2]. In the same year Yamakawa in Japan described the same histopathological findings in temporal bones of patients with the Menière's syndrome [3].

From then on, several temporal bone histopathologists [4–6] found endolymphatic hydrops (EH) in temporal bones of patients with the Menière's syndrome. So, EH was established as the pathological correlate of MD.

Schuknecht [7] in 1978 observed rupture of endolymphatic membranes in patients with EH (**Figures 1** and **2**) in temporal bones of patients who had the Menière's syndrome during their life time. Lawrence in 1864 [8] had shown that rupture of Reisner's membrane in one segment of the chinchilla's cochlear duct and consequent mixing of endolymph with perilymph would cause permanent damage to the organ of Corti in the involved segment.

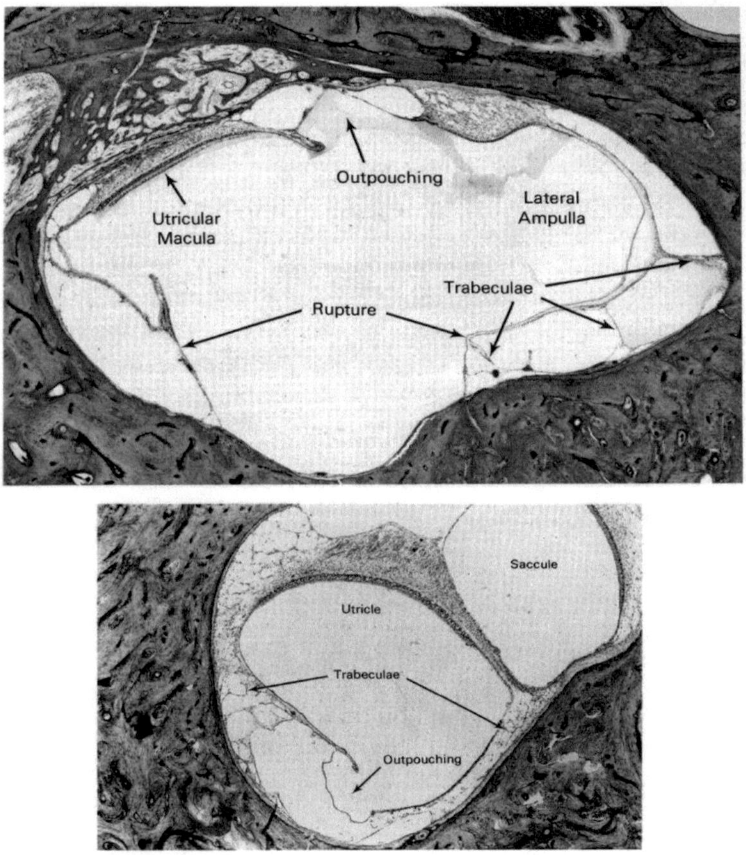

Figure 1.
Membrane rupture in the vestibular labyrinth. Reprinted with permission from Ref. [7].

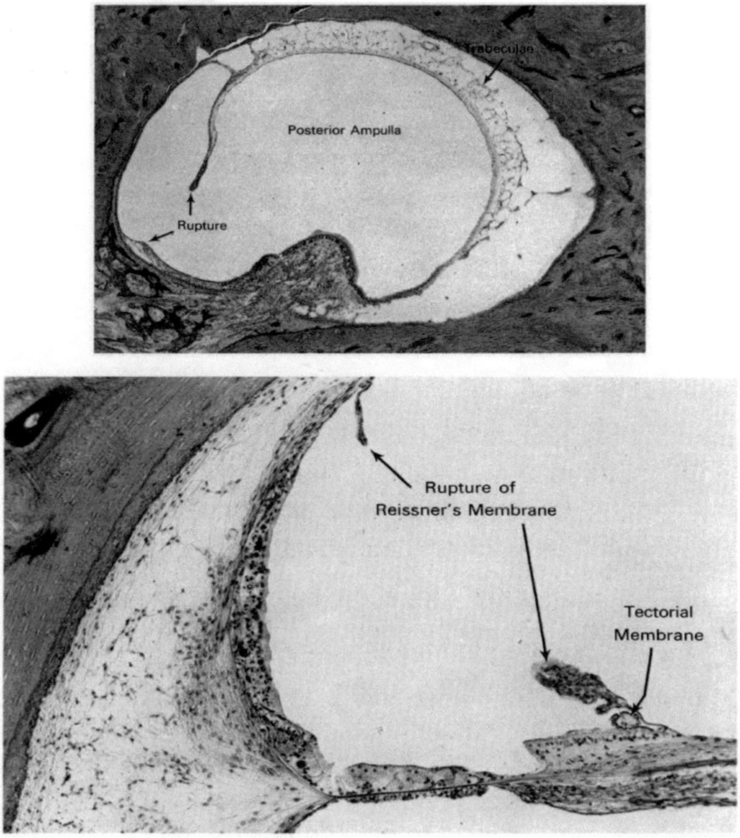

Figure 2.
Membrane ruptures in the semicircular canal and cochlea duct. Reprinted with permission from Ref. [7].

Based on the ruptures of cochlear and vestibular membranes in the hydropic ears Schuknecht proposed that these ruptures and the consequent mixing of endolymph and perilymph would cause the acute Menière's attack.

After the Schuknecht paper EH became more than a pathologic correlate. It was the cause of the Menière's symptoms. For one decade this theory was accepted as true and things appeared to be settled down regarding the etiopathology of Menière's disease.

However, during the year of 1989 Oliveira selected 83 temporal bones of patients who had significant tinnitus during life and tried to find a pathologic correlate for this symptom. Thirty-seven temporal bones had normal histology (44.5%), 23 had EH (27.7%). Among the normal histology bones there were 13 patients who also had episodic vertigo during life. It was notable that 72.2% of the bones had normal histology and EH. He thought of a common cause for MD and EH. In that case EH would not be the cause for MD but both would have a common cause [8].

Rauch et al. in 1989 [9] studied 26 temporal bones from patients who had MD during their life's time but only 13 of them had EH. **Figures 3** and **4** are from Rauch's paper and express the change in position of EH: from the cause of the symptoms to an epiphenomenon also caused by an unknown primary event.

Fraysse in 1990 [10] pointed out that EH may be present in several diseases of the inner ear and that MD patients may not have EH present. Merchant et al. in 1995 found 28 temporal bones from patients with MD who had EH but 19 other patients with EH never had MD symptoms during life [11].

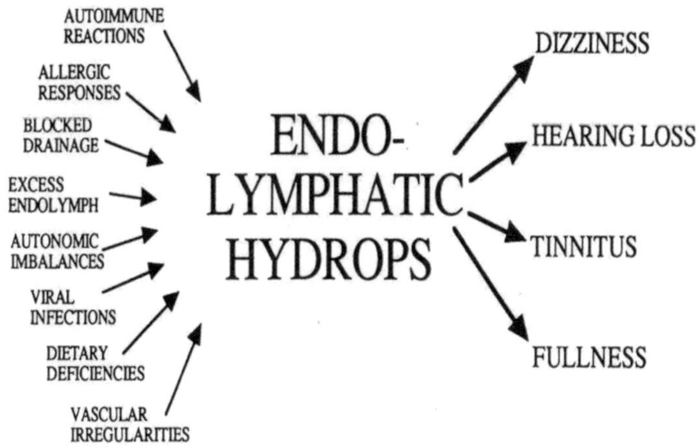

Figure 3.
Reprinted with permission from Ref. [9]. See text for explanation.

In this way the rupture theory put forward by Schuknecht is now discarded. Summarizing what has been said above:

1. EH is present in most cases of MD but it is not the cause of the Menière's symptoms. At most it can be taken as a pathologic correlate for MD. A primary unknown cause produces first the symptoms and later EH as an epiphenomenon.

2. Menière's syndrome is indeed a reaction of the inner ear to many insults (infection, trauma, tertiary syphilis, otosclerosis, autoimmune diseases).

3. EH may be found in the temporal bones from patients with all the above-mentioned insults: it is therefore a common pathologic correlate to many inner ear injuries.

4. We consider as MD the Menière's syndrome without a known cause.

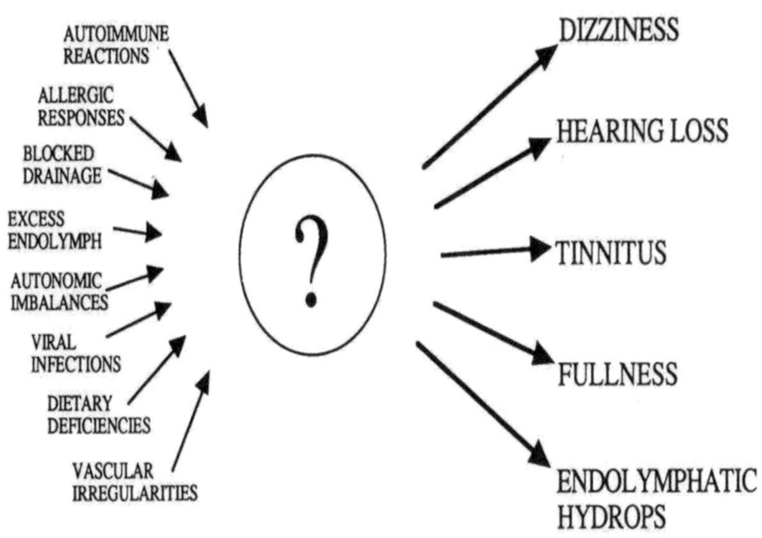

Figure 4.
Reprinted with permission from Ref. [9]. See text for explanation.

2. Familial Menière's disease

Familial MD is not a rare finding. The presence of MD in several siblings of a family points to a genetic etiology for the disease. Studying these families is a way to learn about MD etiology. In this section we will discuss our experience with MD occurring in families.

This research line started up in 1992 [12]. By that time, we saw a patient who was 69 years old and had a full blown Menière's syndrome: severe episodic rotatory vertigo with drop (falling) attacks, tinnitus and fluctuating hearing loss in his right year. These symptoms started up 5 years before we saw him. His drop attacks were severe and several times he hearts himself during falls. Right sided headaches usually preceded the crisis. Audiogram showed low tone sensorineural hearing loss bilateral and flat severe sensorineural hearing loss on the right ear. Left ear had hearing preserved in the frequencies above 500 Hz (**Figure 5A**). VDRL test was negative and glycerol test was positive bilaterally. An endolymphatic sac procedure

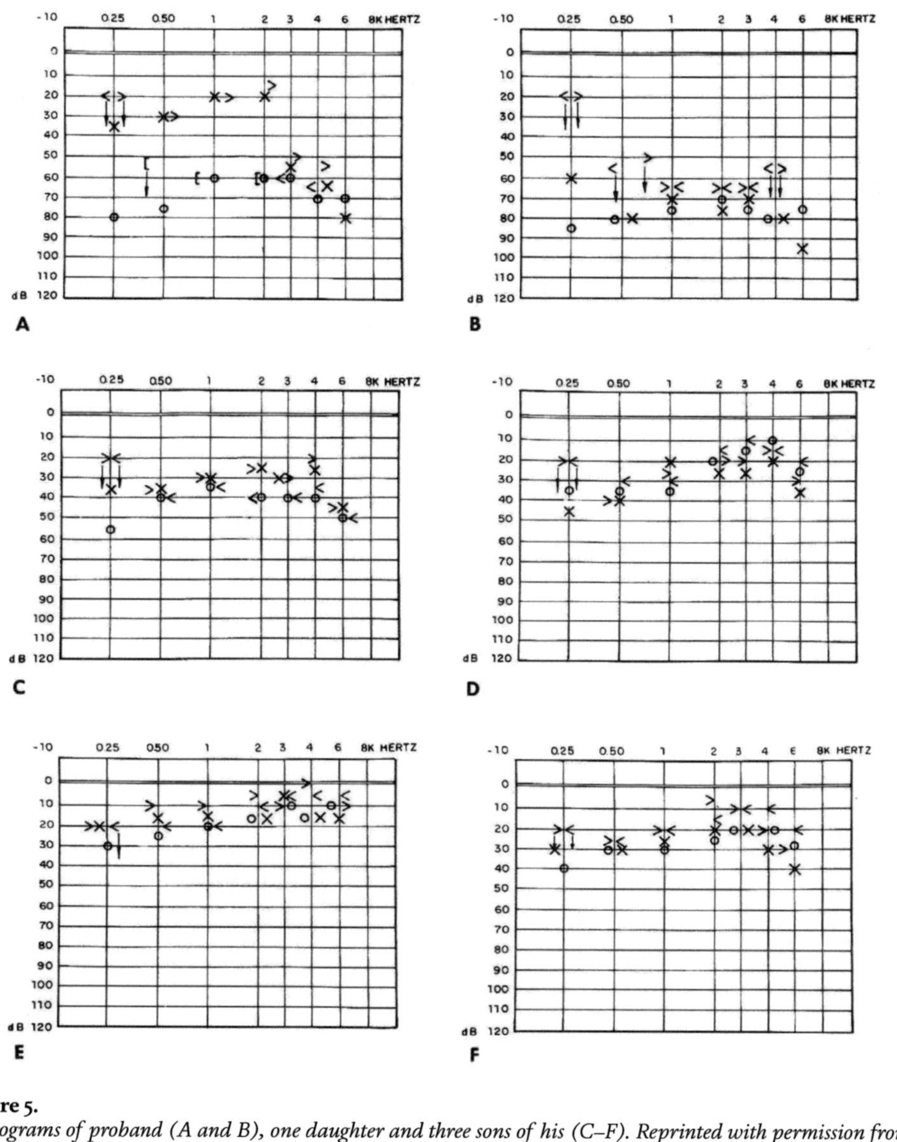

Figure 5.
Audiograms of proband (A and B), one daughter and three sons of his (C–F). Reprinted with permission from Ref. [13].

was performed in his right ear and the drop attacks disappeared. Mild dizziness attacks and headache continued but were controlled on medication. Ten years later in June 1090 his hearing in the right ear had worsened (**Figure 5B**) considerably but the drop attacks had not come back and his dizziness was under control. His headache was unchanged.

The heredogram of this family (**Figure 6**) shows that six of seven sons and daughters of this man had the same complaints as their father and the audiograms on four available siblings showed low tone sensorineural hearing loss (**Figure 5C–F**). One offspring from a second marriage of the index patients also had the same complaints. We did not give attention to the headache these patients complained about so we did not classify this symptom properly.

We found several reports of headache associated with both familial and sporadic Menière's syndrome [13–15] but the headache was not well characterized in any.

Two questions were in our minds after we studied the family described above: (1) how often a family history could be elicited from patients with classic Menière's syndrome; (2) what kind of headache was associated with Menière's syndrome? We started to apply to all the patients with Menière's syndrome seen in our clinic a questionnaire with questions about the presence of similar symptoms in their family members as well as about the presence of migraine symptoms.

Through this questionnaire we identified a large family who had typical Menière's syndrome present in some siblings, migraine and Menière's syndrome in others, and only migraine symptoms in others. Considering all siblings affected with these symptoms we arrived to the heredogram displayed in **Figure 7**. The mode of genetic transmission was clearly autosomal dominant [17]. Of course, we knew that in every day clinic work we find more patients with incomplete than with full blown Menière's syndrome. To consider patients with migraine only as affected siblings was an assumption that was supported by continuing the line of thought.

The summary of all symptoms present on 19 affected members of the family is in **Table 1**. It can be seen there the spectrum of symptoms with some of them present and others absent in different patients. The index patient had full blown Menière's syndrome and fluctuating low tone sensorineural hearing loss (**Figure 8**). Three of his sons had intractable migraine who needed hospitalization for treatment sometimes but they lacked Menière's syndrome symptoms at that point. We concluded that: there was a strong association between migraine and Menière's syndrome in this family and both seemed to be transmitted by a single gene in an autosomal dominant mode. From a physiopathology stand point we do not know how the migraine (central) relates to the Menière's symptoms (peripheral).

Now we had a hypothesis: migraine and Menière's syndrome are related and transmitted in an autosomal dominant mode. To further this hypothesis, we set up to answer two questions: (1) How often is the occurrence of familial

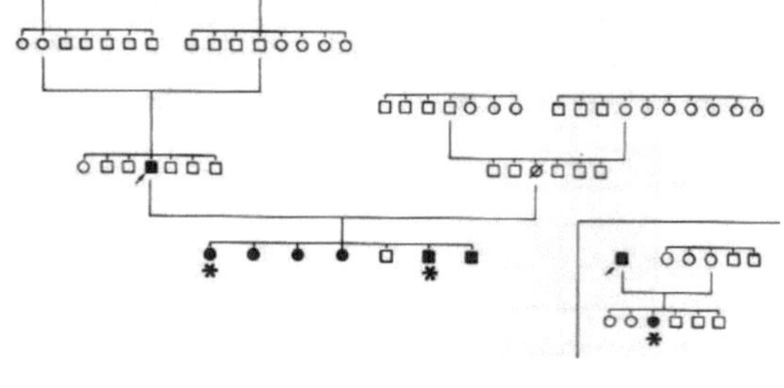

Figure 6.
Heredogram of the 1992 family. Reprinted with permission from Ref. [13]. Black symbols are affected siblings. Circles are male and square are females.

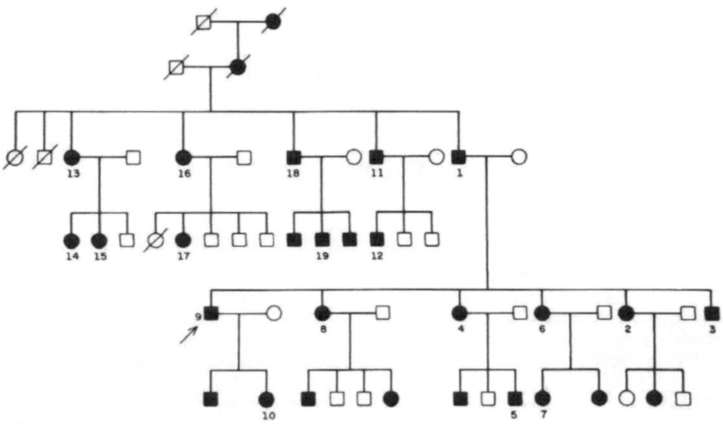

Figure 7.
Heredogram of 1997 family. Reprinted with permission from Ref. [16]. Black symbols are affected siblings. Circles are males and square are females.

Migraine–Menière's syndrome in our population? (2) How is the evolution of these symptoms as time goes by? In other words: what is the Natural History of this symptom's complex?

We then started to apply a questionnaire inquiring about the family history of every patient with typical Menière's syndrome seen in our Otology Clinic prospectively beginning in January 1997 and finishing in December 1998.

All index patients were required to have typical Menière's syndrome according to the American Academy of Otolaryngology—Head and Neck Surgery criteria. The work up included audiometry, tympanometry, vectoeletronystagmography and a glycerol test in order to seal the diagnosis of idiopathic typical Menière's syndrome (Menière's disease). At this point the included patients were questioned about migraine symptoms. Next the questionnaire about their family history regarding Menière's and migraine's symptoms present in other family members was applied. It is worth to mention that any symptom of one of these syndromes were noted and used to construct the heredogram of each family. Every available affected member of these families went through the same work up of the index patients.

Eight patients with typical, complete Menière's syndrome were collected in 2 years from our otology clinic in Brasília. Six of the eight had positive family history for Menière's and/or migraine. **Table 2** shows that only one index patient had low tone sensorineural hearing loss. All others displayed high tone sensorineural hearing loss in between crisis. **Table 3** shows the presence/absence of Menière's and migraine symptoms in the affected members as well as demographic data.

Age of the index patients varied from 26 to 63 years old. Symptoms appeared between 15 and 40 years. Six patients had unilateral symptoms and two had both ears affected. Most of the time migraine occurred before the vestibular symptoms, sometimes it came after the vestibular crisis and a minority had migraine unrelated to the vertiginous attack. In six of the eight indices patient's headache fit the classification of the International Headache Society of 1988 as migraine. There were six female and two male probands [16].

Figures 9–11 show heredograms of the six affected families. It is clear from them that the pattern of genetic transmission is autosomal dominant and there is great variability with some siblings having typical Menière's disease and migraine, others having migraine alone and others having symptoms of Menière's syndrome incomplete with or without migraine. If we assume a monogenetic transmission then variable penetrance of the gene is probably the cause of this variability.

Patient	Age	Sex	Tinnitus	Hearing Loss	Vertigo	Headache	Vomiting	Nausea	Scotomas
1	22	M	+	+	+	–	+	+	–
2	41	F	+	+	+	+*	+	+	+
3	50	M	+	+	+	+*	+	+	+
4	46	F	+	+	+	+*	+	+	+
5	17	M	–	–	–	+*	+	+	+
6	41	F	+	+	+	+	+	+	+
7	19	F	–	–	–	+*	+	+	+
8	56	F	+	–	+	+	–	+	+
9	58	M	+	+	+	+*	+	+	+
10	15	F	+	–	+	+*	+	+	+
11	77	M	+	+	+	–	+	+	–
12	51	M	+	+	+	+*	–	–	+
13	71	F	+	+	+	+	+	+	–
14	49	F	–	–	–	+*	–	–	–
15	47	F	+	+	+	+	–	–	–
16	80	F	+	–	+	+	–	–	–
17	59	F	+	+	+	+*	–	+	+
18	75	M	+	+	+	+	+	+	+
19	45	M	–	–	–	+*	–	–	–

ENG — electronystagmography, N — normal, SNHL — sensorineural hearing loss, ND — not done, MS — Meniere's syndrome, HL — hyperactive labyrinth.

*Headache was described by patient as typical migraine.

Patient	Anopsia	Paresthesia	Age (y) at Which Symptoms Appeared	Time Sequence of Headache and Vertigo	Blood Tests	Audiometry	Tympanometry	ENG
1	+	–	30		N	SNHL, bilateral, down-sloping	N	ND
2	+	–	10	Headache precedes vertigo	ND	ND	ND	ND
3	–	–	10	Variable	ND	ND	ND	ND
4	–	+	13 migraine, 30 MS	Migraine only for 17 years, MS only afterward	N	Mild SNHL, bilateral, 500 and 1,000 Hz	N	N
5	+	–	15		ND	Mild SNHL, bilateral, 500 and 1,000 Hz	ND	N
6	–	+	14	Headache precedes vertigo	N	Bilateral moderate SNHL, down-sloping	N	HL left side
7	–	–	10		ND	ND	N	N
8	+	+	9	Headache and scotomas precede vertigo	N	Mild SNHL, 500 and 1,000 Hz, right	N	HL left side
9	–	–	39	Headache precedes vertigo	N	Bilateral moderate SNHL, down-sloping	N	HL left side
10	–	–	7	Headache precedes vertigo	ND	ND	ND	ND
11	–	–	18		ND	Bilateral moderate SNHL, down-sloping	N	HL left side
12	+	–	17 migraine, 25 MS	Migraine only for 8 years, then MS only	ND	Bilateral moderate SNHL, down-sloping	N	HL bilateral
13	–	–	30	Variable	N	Bilateral mixed hearing loss, worse on left	ND	HL bilateral
14	–	–	20		ND	ND	ND	ND
15	–	–	35	Variable	N	Mild SNHL, left	N	HL bilateral
16	–	–	21	Variable	ND	ND	ND	ND
17	+	+	43	Variable	ND	ND	ND	ND
18	–	–	15	Headache precedes vertigo	ND	ND	ND	ND
19	–	–	20		ND	ND	ND	ND

ENG — electronystagmography, N — normal, SNHL — sensorineural hearing loss, ND — not done, MS — Meniere's syndrome, HL — hyperactive labyrinth.

*Headache was described by patient as typical migraine.

* *Reprinted with permission from Ref. [16].*

Table 1.
*Summary of clinical, laboratory, audiometric, and electronystagmographic findings in 19 affected members of family studied in 1997.**

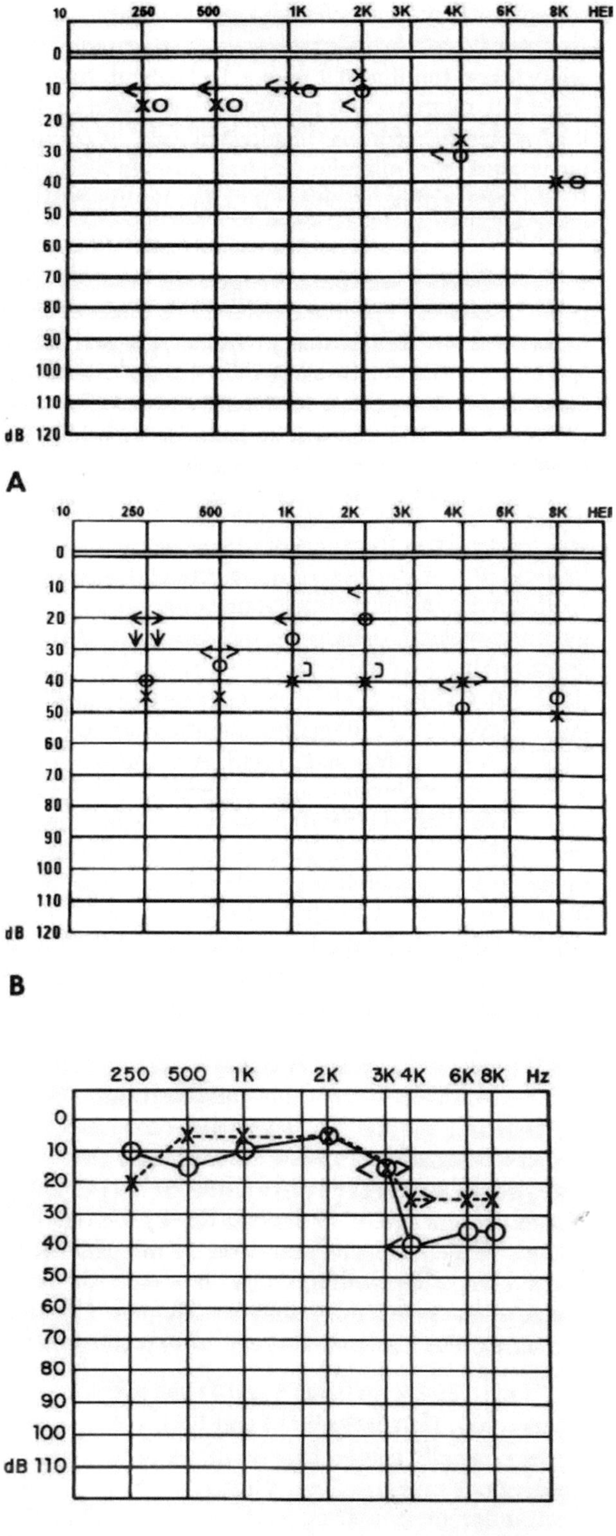

Figure 8.
Audiograms of the proband of the 1997 family. (A–C) Document fluctuating low tones sensorineural hearing loss. Reprinted with permission from Ref. [16].

Proband	Age (y)	Sex	Audiometry
1	62	M	Bilateral moderate SNHL, downsloping on R, flat on L
2	43	F	Bilateral downsloping SNHL, moderate on R, severe on L
3	30	F	Normal
4	46	F	Normal
5	43	F	Flat moderate SNHL on R, normal on L
6	26	F	Normal
7	45	M	Bilateral moderate SNHL low and high tones, worse on L, middle tones normal
8	35	F	Moderate low-tone SNHL on L, normal on R

Speech discrimination score was compatible with pure tone loss in all patients.

SNHL — sensorineural hearing loss.

Reprinted with permission from Ref. [18].

Table 2.
*Summary of audiometric findings in eight probands (2002 paper).**

Probands	Affected Family Members	Age (y)	Sex	Tinnitus	Aural Fullness	Fluctuating Hearing Loss	Vertigo	Nausea	Vomiting	Audiometry	VENG	Scotoma	Photophobia	Atypical Headache	Hemicranial Headache	Pulsatile Headache
III-5		30	F	+	+	+	+	+	+	N	PIS R	+	+	–	+	+
(Family 3)	I -2	Deceased	F	+	+	+	+	+	–	ND	ND	+	+	–	+	+
	II-2	60	F	–	–	–	–	+	–	ND	ND	+	+	–	+	+
	III-6	16	F	+	–	+	+	–	–	SNHL bilat	PIS R	+	+	–	+	+
	III-8	37	F	–	–	–	–	+	–	ND	ND	–	+	–	+	+
	IV-1	10	M	+	+	+	+	–	–	N	N	–	–	+	–	–
III-2		46	F	+	+	+	+	+	+	N	PIS R	–	–	+	–	–
(Family 4)	II-2	60	F	+	–	–	+	–	–	N	N	–	+	–	+	+
	II-3	58	F	+	–	–	+	–	–	N	N	+	–	–	+	+
	II-4	65	F	+	+	–	+	+	+	N	PIS L	–	+	–	+	+
	III-3	43	F	–	–	–	+	–	–	N	PIS bilat	+	+	–	+	+
	III-7	33	F	–	–	–	–	–	–	ND	ND	–	+	–	+	+
	III-8	32	F	–	–	–	–	–	+	ND	ND	–	+	–	–	–
	IV-1	25	F	–	–	–	+	+	–	ND	ND	–	–	–	–	–
III-5		43	F	+	+	+	+	+	+	SNHL R	ND	+	+	–	+	+
(Family 5)	III-4	46	F	+	–	–	+	–	–	N	N	–	–	+	–	–
	IV-3	14	F	+	–	+	–	–	–	N	N	–	–	–	–	–
III-9		26	F	+	+	+	+	+	+	N	PIS bilat	+	+	–	+	+
(Family 6)	II-5	75	M	+	–	–	+	+	+	SNHL L	N	–	+	–	+	+
	III-8	32	F	+	–	–	+	–	–	ND	ND	–	+	–	+	+
	II-4	65	F	–	–	–	–	+	–	ND	ND	–	+	–	+	+
	III-2	46	M	–	–	–	–	–	–	ND	ND	–	+	–	–	–
	III-6	36	F	–	–	–	+	+	–	ND	ND	–	+	–	+	+
	II-1	40	F	–	–	–	–	+	–	ND	ND	+	+	–	+	–
	II-2	50	F	–	–	–	–	–	–	ND	ND	+	–	–	+	+
	II-4	52	F	–	–	–	–	+	+	ND	ND	–	+	–	+	+
II-22		45	M	+	+	+	+	+	+	SNHL L	N	–	–	–	–	–
(Family 7)	II-13	62	M	+	+	–	+	+	–	SNHL bilat	ND	+	–	+	+	+
	II-18	58	M	–	–	+	+	–	–	SNHL bilat	ND	–	–	–	–	–
	II-17	56	F	+	–	+	–	–	–	SNHL bilat	ND	+	–	+	+	+
	III-4	20	F	+	+	+	–	–	–	ND	ND	–	+	–	+	+
	III-5	12	F	–	–	–	–	–	–	N	N	–	+	–	+	+
III-5		35	F	+	+	+	+	+	+	N	PIS bilat	+	+	–	+	+
(Family 8)	II-5	54	F	+	–	+	–	+	–	ND	ND	+	+	–	+	+
	II-1	50	F	–	–	–	+	+	–	ND	ND	–	–	–	+	+

Tympanometric and stapedial reflex results were normal in all patients who had them done. Proband 1 had full-blown Meniere's syndrome and atypical headache. Proband 2 had both Meniere's and migraine symptoms.

VENG — vectoelectronystagmography, N — normal, PIS — peripheral irritative syndrome, ND — not done.

** Reprinted with permission from Ref. [18].*

Table 3.
*Summary of clinical, audiometric, and VENG findings in affected members of six families.**

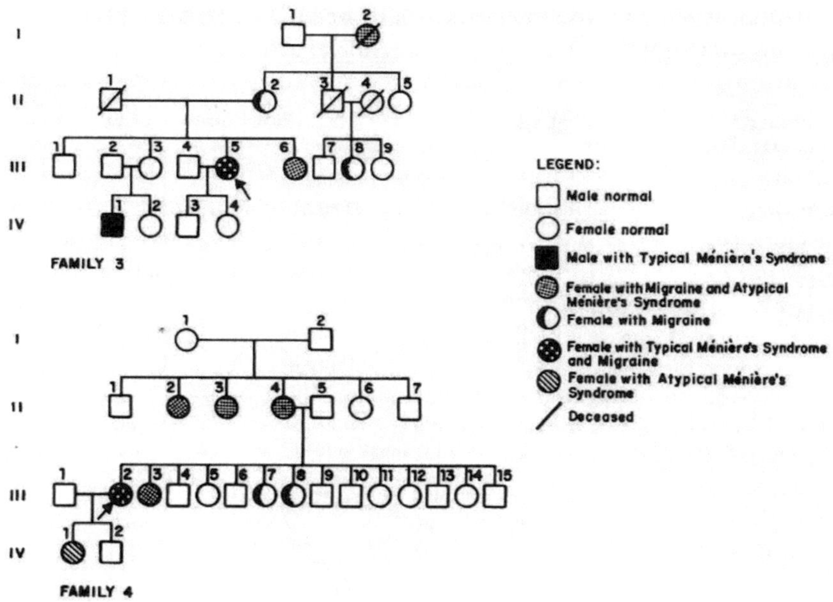

Figure 9.
Heredograms of families 3 and 4 from the 2002 paper. Note the spectrum of migraine and Menière's syndrome present in the affected siblings. Reprinted with permission from Ref. [18].

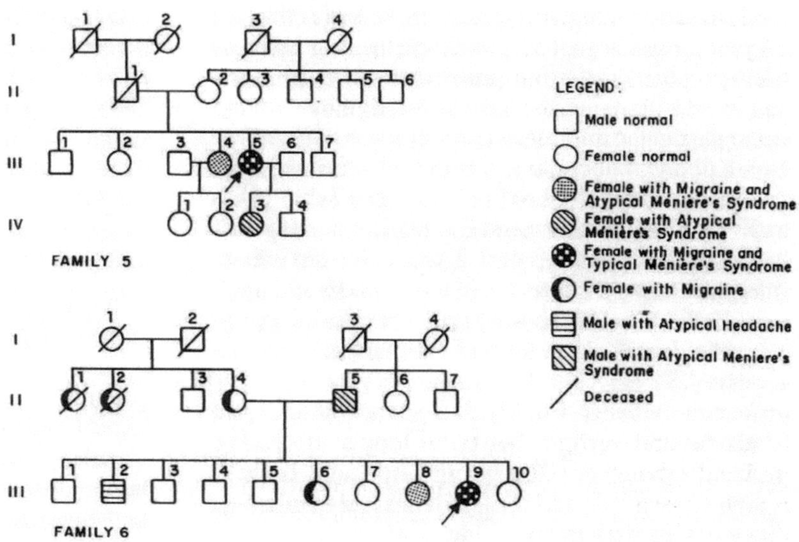

Figure 10.
Heredograms of families 5 and 6 of the 2002 paper. The pattern of symptoms distribution among the siblings are similar to the one present in families 3 and 4 above. Reprinted with permission from Ref. [18].

From these data we reasoned that:

1. Typical Menière's syndrome is not very frequent in Brasília: during 2 years in a very buzzy Otology Clinic we collected only eight cases.

2. On the other hand, the occurrence of familial disease in patients with typical Menière's syndrome (Menière's disease) is quite high (six of eight index

patients). If we consider Menière's syndrome all the spectrum of symptoms seen in these families then the disease is not so infrequent. In other words, we see incomplete Menière's syndrome much more often in our clinics than the typical syndrome. However, migraine can be associated with all the Menière`s spectrum of symptoms.

We wanted to ask: what happens to this spectrum of symptoms as time goes by?

The family we published in 1997 [17] lived in Brasília and we were able to follow them up from 1995 on for 10 years. The following paragraphs will refer to unpublished data from our group.

All affected and unaffected siblings in the heredogram in **Figure 7** were carefully interviewed along the 10 years follow up. Twenty siblings had no qualitative changes in symptoms from 1995 to 2005. Four had changed from atypical headache in 1995 to typical migraine 10 years later. Two had migraine in 1995 and progressed to Menière's syndrome in 2005. Four siblings had vertigo and atypical headache in 1995 and progressed to vertigo and typical migraine in 2005.

Five unaffected siblings in 1995 had symptoms of the migraine—Menière's complex 10 years later: two with aural fullness, one with migraine, tinnitus, vertigo and hearing loss and two with migraine and vertigo. Three affected siblings had remarkable improvement in migraine and vertigo or complete remission of the symptoms.

Fifteen of the 38 affected siblings started out with migraine and the vestibular symptoms appeared in average 17.6 years later. Seven siblings continued with migraine only after 10 years follow up. Over time the intensity and periodicity of the migraine symptoms tended to diminish and the vestibular symptoms tended to become more frequent and intense (**Table 4** and **Figure 12**).

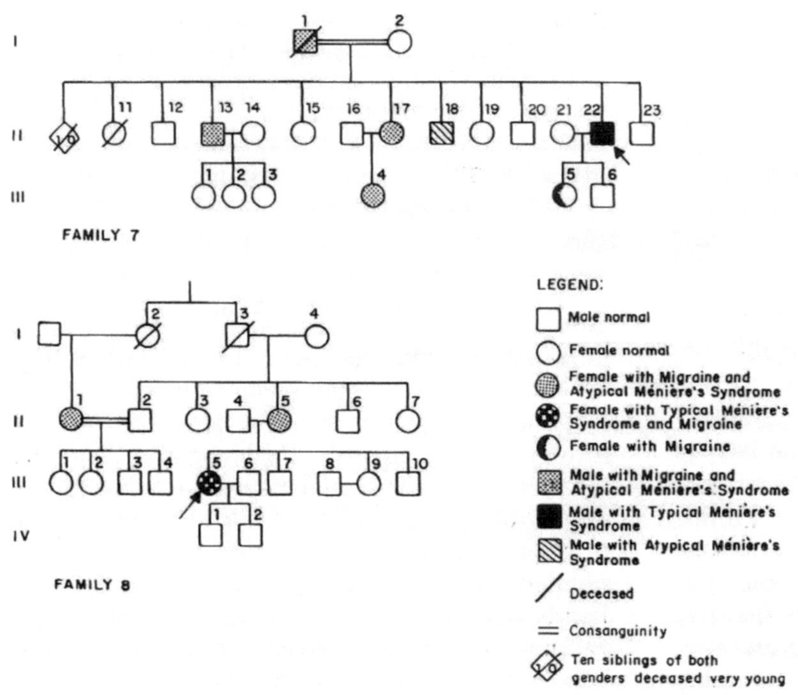

Figure 11.
Heredogram of families 7 and 8 of the 2002 paper. The pattern of symptoms among the siblings is similar to the families 3to 6. Reprinted with permission from Ref. [18].

Patient	Age at the moment (2005) (y)	Periodicity* (1995)		Periodicity* (2005)		Intensity (1995)		Intensity (2005)	
		Migraine	Menière	Migraine	Menière	Migraine	Menière	Migraine	Menière
1	81	2/w	1/w	1/w	1/w	9/10	Moderate	6/10	Severe
2	90	—	—	—	—	—	—	—	—
3	82	2/w	2/m	2/m	1/w	8/10	Moderate	6/10	Severe
4	87	1/w	1/m	1/m	1/w	6/10	Moderate	6/10	Severe
5	92	1/w	1/w	2/m	2/w	9/10	Severe	9/10	Severe
11	62	2/m	—	2/m	1/m	8/10	—	7/10	Severe
12	58	2/m	—	2/m	—	7/10	—	6/10	—
21	69	1/m	1/m	1/m	2/m	8/10	Moderate	5/10	Moderate
31	61	1/m	1/m	1/m	2/m	9/10	Moderate	6/10	Moderate
32	64	3–4/m	—	2/m	—	9/10	—	6/10	—
33	63	1/m	—	1/m	—	10/10	—	6/10	—
41	61	2/w	1/w	2/m	2/w	9/10	Moderate	7/10	Severe
51	68	1/m	1/m	1/m	2/m	9/10	Severe	8/10	Severe
52	66	1/m	—	1/m	—	8/10	—	8/10	—
53	54	1/m	2/y	1/m	4/y	7/10	Moderate	7/10	Severe
54	51	2/y	3/y	2/y	1/m	8/10	Moderate	8/10	Moderate
55	51	3/y	1/y	3/y	3/y	8/10	Moderate	6/10	Moderate
56	60	1/m	2/y	1/m	1/m	9/10	Moderate	8/10	Moderate
512	37	6/y	1/y	2/m	4/y	8/10	Moderate	8/10	Moderate
524	37	1/m	—	1/m	—	8/10	—	8/10	—
531	32	3/y	—	3/y	—	7/10	—	7/10	—
533	25	3/y	—	3/y	—	7/10	—	7/10	—
541	29	4/y	1/y	1/m	4/y	8/10	Moderate	8/10	Moderate

Unpublished observations.

Table 4.
*Natural history of migraine and vestibular symptoms during 10 years follow-up (1997 family) (N = 23 affected siblings).**

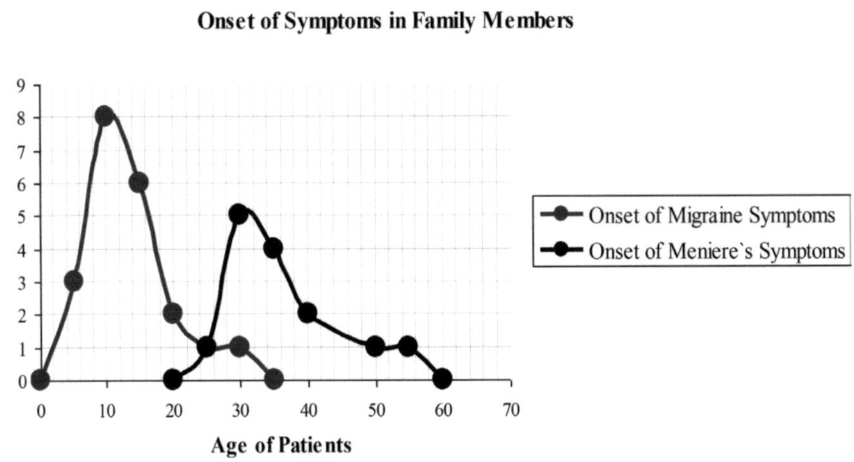

Figure 12.
Graphic representation of the natural history of this symptom complex during 10 years follow up of the 1997 family.

Patient	Audiogram result (1995)	Audiogram result (2005)
1	Moderate to profound mixed hearing loss bilaterally	Profound mixed hearing loss bilaterally
2	Mild high frequency SNHL	Mild to moderate high frequency SNHL
3	Moderate high frequency SNHL	Moderate high frequency SNHL
4	Moderate mixed hearing loss bilaterally	Moderate mixed hearing loss bilaterally
5	Moderate high frequency SNHL bilaterally	Moderate to severe high frequency SNHL bilaterally
11	Normal	Normal
12	Normal	Normal
13	—	—
21	Normal	Normal
22	—	—
23	—	—
24	—	—
31	—	—
32	Normal	Mild high frequency SNHL bilaterally
33	—	—
41	Mild high frequency SNHL	Mild to moderate high frequency SNHL bilaterally
42	—	—
43	—	—
51	Moderate high frequency SNHL bilaterally	Profound high frequency SNHL bilaterally
52	Normal	Normal
53	Normal	Normal
54	Mild high frequency SNHL bilaterally	Mild to moderate high frequency SNHL bilaterally
55	Mild high frequency SNHL bilaterally	Mild to moderate high frequency SNHL bilaterally
56	Moderate high frequency SNHL	Profound high frequency SNHL bilaterally

Patient	Audiogram result (1995)	Audiogram result (2005)
511	—	—
512	Normal	Mild high frequency SNHL bilaterally
521	—	—
522	—	—
523	—	—
524	—	—
531	—	—
532	—	—
533	Normal	Normal
541	Normal	Normal
542	—	—
551	—	—
552	—	—
553	—	—

**Reprinted with permission from Ref. [19].*

Table 5.
*Hearing loss during 10 years follow-up (N = 19).**

Hearing loss worsened in most patients. The loss was in high frequency tones and bilateral (**Table 5**). We were not able to document low tone fluctuating sensorineural hearing loss during the crisis of vertigo/migraine in all siblings but we did document this feature clearly only in the index patient (**Figure 8**).

Now we had the natural history of this complex of symptoms described. We were therefore able to organize the clinical data in order to define a phenotype of this syndrome in the large family from Brasília.

Our hypothesis was that this was a genetically determined symptom complex and the genetic transmission was monogenic with incomplete penetrance. Next step was to try to find the genetic locus for these symptoms. Because we were not able to document low tone sensorineural hearing loss in most of the siblings and the high frequency sensorineural hearing loss was bilateral in the majority of the siblings the clinical diagnosis of migrainous vertigo was adopted for these patients. The fact that some of them had typical Menière's syndrome including low tone sensorineural hearing loss was however pointed out in the final paper [18].

Twenty-three family members who were clinically and audiologically evaluated and had image studies also done had genome wide linkage analysis performed with Affymetrix GeneChip Human Mapping 10K microarrays. Genotyping of family members DNA with microsatellite markers was used to further assess candidate loci identified from the whole genome scan.

The results of vestibular testing and imaging studies were unremarkable. The genetic analysis defined a 12.0 MB interval on chromosome 5q35 between loci rs2448795 and D5S2073 that contained the disease gene (logarithm of odd score 4.21).

Molecular genetics studies were performed at the Molecular Genetics laboratory of Harvard Medical School headed by Professor Jonathan Seidman.

3. Discussion of above findings and correlation with current literature

Here we will blend our results with the current literature on the subject and formulate a new hypothesis.

It is important to acknowledge the recently described vertiginous migraine (VM) syndrome [19] which is now listed in the Barany Society and the International Headache Society classification of vestibular diseases [20]. This entity is very frequent, second only to benign paroxistic positional vertigo being probably present in 1% of the general population [8]. We are not going to describe in detail the VM symptoms but it is important to point out the differences between MD and VM.

One marked difference is the absence of hearing loss that fluctuates in the low frequencies in the beginning and that progresses to severe hearing loss along the life in Menière's disease but not in vertiginous migraine. Bilaterally of the symptoms seems to be more frequent in familial MD and VM than in sporadic MD but it is not different between these two syndromes.

There is a significant body of literature dealing with the interfaces of Menière's disease (DM) and VM. We will review briefly some papers on this subject.

Neuhauser et al. [21, 22] prospectively evaluated migraine in 200 patients from a dizziness clinic and 200 ones from a migraine clinic. Prevalence of migraine that satisfied the criteria of the International Headache Society (HIS) II was 38% in the dizziness clinic and 24% in sex and age matched controls ($p < 0.01$). Vertiginous migraine was present in 7% of patients in the dizziness clinic and 9% of the ones in the migraine clinic. In 15 of 32 patient's vertigo was always associated with migraine during the acute attacks. In 16 patients this association was sporadic and two patients never had both symptoms together.

Radke et al. [23] studied 78 patients (40 male and 38 female) aged 29–81 years all with idiopathic uni- or bilateral Menière's disease according to the AAO-HNS criteria. Lifetime prevalence of migraine with and without aura was 50% among these patients and 25% among normal control patients ($p < 0.001$). Furthermore 45% or the Menière's disease patients always experienced at least one migraine symptom (headache, photophobia, aura) during the acute attacks. They postulated a pathophysiologic link between migraine and MD.

Urkur et al. [24] studied VEMPs parameters in VM, MD and migraine patients and found very similar results for all these patients. Gazques et al. [13] published a paper on recent advances in the genetics of recurrent vertigo including familiar episodic ataxias and MD. They found that 20% of MD patients have positive family histories for this disease [25].

Cha et al. [27] described six families with index patients affected by MD and migraine. There were 56 affected siblings. Of these 26 (41%) met the HIS criteria for migraine. Fifty percent had migraine with aura. Three patients had typical aura without headache. Sixty-three family members had recurrent spells of spontaneous vertigo. There were three twin pairs, two monos and one dizygotic. One of the homozygotic pair had migraine and MD while the other one had migraine and episodic vertigo without auditory involvement (VM).

Bertora and Bergman [38] using quantitative EEG (qEEG) studied 120 patients with MD and migraine and 85 patients with MD and no migraine. Eighty-five percent of MDs patients had hemodynamic brain variations like the ones found in migraine. Brain electric depolarizations and cortical irritative focuses are common to migraine and MD. However, MDs patients had important hyperactivity in the limbic lobe [28].

From this brief review of literature, we can say:

1. VM and MD are very often present in one single family and therefore have a common-genetic link.

2. Hearing involvement in MD and not in VM is the main clinical difference between these two syndromes.

3. Migraine is present in both syndromes.

Recently Welfang et al. [29] selected 30 classic MD patients and 30 patients with definite or probable VM matched by age and sex. Three-dimensional real inversion recovery magnetic resonance (3D real IR) was performed in these patients 24 hours after intratympanic gadolinium injection in order to assess endolymphatic hydrops (EH). Response rates, amplitudes, latency and response thresholds of cervical and ocular evoked myogenic potentials (c/o VEMP) were tested using air conducted sound. Pure tone audiometry was used to evaluate the level of hearing loss.

Different degrees of EH were observed in the cochlea and vestibule of MD patients. Some VM patients had 3D real—IR suspicious for cochlea EH and no EH was found in the vestibule of these patients. There was statistically significant correlation between EH and low tone sensorineural hearing loss. Response thresholds for c/o VEMP were no different in VM and MD patients.

Therefore, low frequencies sensorineural hearing loss correlate with EH on MD patients. 3R-real IR showed more severe degrees of EH in patients with MD but suggestion of EH in the cochlea of VM patients was showed. MD and VM patients behaved similarly in vestibular dysfunction and their transduction pathway (VEMP).

Ghawany et al. [30] treated 25 patients with typical MD following protocol to prophylactic migrainous treatment and showed marked improvement in quality of life in 92% of the patients. He states his results point to etiopathogenetic relation between MD and VM.

These results suggest a common etiopathogenesis for MD and VM and that VM may progress to MD as time goes by if EH develops in VM patients.

4. Conclusion

At this point we know that the spectrum of symptoms that goes from migraine alone to migraine with full blown MD including vertigo and migraine (VM), vertigo alone (atypical Menière's syndrome) has high familial incidence and is genetically transmitted in a monogenic autosomal dominant mode [16]. We have found that the locus for this spectrum of symptoms maps to chromosome 5q35 [18].

Studies using VEMP [26] and 3D real IR [27] have shown that EH is present in different degrees in both MD and VM. It may be that absence of low tone sensorineural hearing loss in VM relates to the very small degree of EH present in this entity compared to MD.

Based on all this evidence we have up to now we believe that future efforts should be directed to isolate the gene in chromosome 5q35 and follow up longitudinally patients with VM with VEMP and 3D real IR MRI to test the hypothesis that VM and MD are different stages of the same process.

Sporadic MD and VM should be tested for the presence of the gene we are looking for after we have it isolated. Then we might also have a better idea about the etiology of MD and VM. Probably environmental factors [31] will be also important for the full development of the disease (multifactorial etiology).

We do believe that this research line should be taken to its future.

5. Etiopathogenesis of migraine—Menière's disease

Finally we must consider how migraine, a central syndrome relates to Meniere's disease a syndrome that originates in the periphery of the vestibular system.

Several authors [32–36] have shown that trigeminal vasomotor fibers innervate the inner ear (stria vascularis, cells of the ampullary crests) and through this pathway the vascular changes occurring in the central nervous system reach the peripheric vestibular system and bring about the symptoms of MD and EH. This certainly would occur in VM too.

Of course this theory needs experimental confirmation before it can be considered proven. Nevertheless the anatomical pathways are in existence and this is factual evidence towards this theory. The natural history of the symptoms in our families supports it.

Dolowitz [37] has studied a big number of patients with MD and showed that headache is a nuclear symptom in sporadic MD but he did not characterize the headache as igraine so this must be done before we can say that migraine is a constant part of sporadic MD.

Author details

Carlos A. Oliveira
Brasília University Medical School, Brasília, DF, Brazil

*Address all correspondence to: cacpoliveira@brturbo.com.br

References

[1] Menière P. Memoires sur dês lesions de l`òreille interne donnant lieu a dês symptoms de congestion cerebrale apoplectiforme. GazMedicale de Paris. 1861;**15**:597-601

[2] Hallpike LS, Cairns H. Observations on the pathology of Meniere's syndrome. The Journal of Laryngology and Otology. 1938;**53**:625-655

[3] Yamakaua KJ. Pathologic changes in a Meniere's patient. Journal of Otolaryngology Society of Japan. 1938:2310-2312

[4] Hallpike LS, Wright HS. Histological findings in case of Menière's disease with remarks on pathologic anatomy and basis of this lesion. The Journal of Laryngology and Otology. 1940;**55**:59-66

[5] Lindsay JR. Histological studies of Menière's disease. Archives of Otolaryngology. 1994;**37**:853-867

[6] Altman F, Kornfeld M. LXXV histological studies of Meniere's disease. The Annals of Otology, Rhinology, & Laryngology. 1965;**74**:935-943

[7] Schuknecht HF. A critical evaluation of treatment for Meniere's disease. Journal of Contact Rd ORL Allergy. 1978;**40**:15-30

[8] Fraysse BG, Alonso A, House WF. Observations on the pathology of Meniere's syndrome. Annals of Otology, Rhinology and Laryngology. 1980;**89**(Suppl 6):2-22

[9] Rauch SD, Merchant SN, Thedinger BA. Menière's syndrome and endolymphatic hydrops. The Annals of Otology, Rhinology, and Laryngology. 1989;**98**:873-883

[10] HYS K. In: Nadol JB, editor. Second International Symposium on Meniere's Disease. Amsterdam: Kugler and Ghedini; 1989

[11] Merchant SN, Adams J, Nadol JB Jr. Pathophysiology of Menière's syndrome: Are symptoms caused by endolymphatic hydrops? Otology & Neurotology. 2005;**26**:74-81

[12] Oliveira CA. Thinking about tinnitus. The International Tinnitus Journal. 1995;**1**:1-4

[13] Oliveira CA, Braga AM. Meniere's syndrome inherited as an autosomal dominant trait. The Annals of Otology, Rhinology, and Laryngology. 1992;**101**:590-594

[14] Brown MR. Meniere's syndrome. Archives of Neurology and Psychiatry. 1941;**46**:561-565

[15] Brown MR. The factor of heredity in labyrinthine deafness and paroxysmal vertigo (Menière's syndrome). The Annals of Otology, Rhinology, and Laryngology. 1949;**58**:665-670

[16] Oliveira CA, Bezerra RL, Araujo MF, Almeida VF, Messias CI. Meniere's syndrome and migraine: Incidence in one family. The Annals of Otology, Rhinology, and Laryngology. 1997;**106**:823-829

[17] Bernstein JM. Occurrence of episodic vertigo and hearing loss in families. The Annals of Otology, Rhinology, and Laryngology. 1965;**74**:1011-1021

[18] Oliveira CA, Messias CI, Ferrari I. Occurrence of familial Meniere's syndrome and migraine in Brasília. 2002;**111**:229-236

[19] Bahmad F Jr, De Palma SR, Merchant SN, Bezerra RL, Oliveira CA, Seidman ES, et al. Locus for familial

migrainous vertigo disease maps to chromosome 5q35. The Annals of Otology, Rhinology, and Laryngology. 2009;**118**:670-676

[20] Neuhauser H, Lempert T. Vestibular migraine. Neurologic Clinics. 2009;**27**(2):379-391

[21] Neuhauser H, Leopold M, von Brevern M, Arnold G, Lempert T. The interrelations of migraine, vertigo and migrainous vertigo. Neurology. 2001;**56**(4):436-441

[22] Lempert T, Olesen JF, Urlan J, Waterson J, Seemungal B, Carey J, et al. Vestibular migraine: Diagnostic criteria. Journal of Vestibular Research. 2012;**22**(4):167-172

[23] Radke A, Lempert T, Gresty MA, Brookes GB, Bronstein AM, Migraine NH. Meniére's disease: Is there a link? Neurology. 2002;**50**(11):1700-1704

[24] Urkur et al. Migrainous vertigo, Manière's disease and migraine. The Journal of International Advanced Otology. 2003;**9**(3):350-367

[25] Oliveira CA. Editorial. The International Tinnitus Journal. 2014;**19**:2-3

[26] Gazques I, Lopes Escames JA. Genetics of recurrent vertigo and vestibular disorders. Genomics. 2011;**12**(6):443-450

[27] Cha HI, Kane MJ, Baloh RHF. Familial clustering of migraine, episodic vertigo and Meniere's disease. Otology & Neurotology. 2008;**29**(1):93-96

[28] Oliveira CA. Letter to the editor. The International Tinnitus Journal. 2017;**21**(76)

[29] Welfang S, Guo P, Rent T, Wanda G. Magnetic resonance imaging of intratympanic gadolinium helps differentiate vestibular migraine from Meniere's disease. Laryngoscope. 2017;**127**:2382-2388

[30] Ghawani Y, Haiden YM, Moshtaghi O, Lin HW, Djalilian HD. Evaluating quality of life in patients with Meniere's disease treated as migraine. The Annals of Otology, Rhinology, and Laryngology. 2018;**125**:877-887

[31] Oniki J, Takahashi M, Wada R, Sato R. Comparative study of the daily lifestyle of patients with Meniere's disease and controls. The Annals of Otology, Rhinology, and Laryngology. 2005;**114**(12):927-933

[32] William HC. A review of the literature as to the physiologic dysfunction of Meniere's disease: A new hypothesis as to its fundamental cause. Laryngoscope. 1965;**75**:1661-1669

[33] Torok M. Etiology as a guide in the management of Menière's disease. Laryngoscope. 1982;**92**:237-238

[34] Vass Z, Steyger PI, Hordichok AJ, Taune DR, Jansen D, Nuttal AL. Capsaicin stimulation of the cochlea and electric stimulation of the trigeminal ganglion mediate vascular permeability in cochlear and vertebra-basilar arteries: A possible cause of inner ear dysfunction in headache. Neuroscience. 2001;**103**:189-201

[35] Vass Z, Shore SE, Nuttal AL, Miller JM. Endolymphatic hydrops reduces retrograde labeling of trigeminal innervations to the cochlea. Experimental Neurology. 1998;**151**:241-248

[36] Pondugula ST, Sanneman JD, Wangemann P, Milhaud Marcus DC. Glucocorticoids stimulates cation absorption by semicircular canal duct epithelium via epithelial sodium channel PG. American Journal of Physiology. Renal Physiology. 2004;**286**:1127-1135

[37] Dolowitz DA. Menière's—An inner ear seizure. Laryngoscope. 1979;**89**:67-77

[38] Bertora GO, Bergman JM. Menière's disease: Is it a special sort of migraine? Our experience. Archives of Sensology and Neurootology in Science and Practice. 2015. Available from: http://www.neurootology.otg/proceedings

Section 3

Nonsurgical Treatment

Chapter 3

Meniere's Disease: Nonsurgical Treatment

Yetkin Zeki Yilmaz, Begum Bahar Yilmaz
and Aysegul Batioglu-Karaaltın

Abstract

Meniere's disease or syndrome is one of the most common inner ear diseases. Meniere's disease is characterized by episodic vertigo, sensorineural hearing loss that fluctuates during episodes, tinnitus, and ear fullness. Ideal treatment should stop vertigo attacks, restore hearing, get rid of tinnitus and ear fullness. Treatment options are decided upon the remaining hearing, severity, and intensity of vertigo attacks. Meniere's disease is progressive on hearing levels of the patient; some of them develop profound hearing loss that also could affect the other ear. In order to plan a treatment scheme for patient, these conditions should be assessed. It has a destructive and progressive nature, so the first step of treatment should contain more conservative treatment options. If symptom control could not be obtained, destructive treatment options should be considered.

Keywords: Meniere's disease, lifestyle changes, Meniett, vestibular rehabilitation, neuro-otology

1. Introduction

Meniere's disease was first described by Prosper Meniere in 1861 [1]. He described series of symptoms of a leukemic patient, and he suggested that vertiginous symptoms were caused by hemorrhage in the inner ear [2]. Knapp hypothesized inner ear hydrops, but its histologic confirmation was demonstrated in 1938 [3]. Still today, Meniere's disease etiology is not clear.

Meniere's disease is characterized by episodic vertigo, sensorineural hearing loss that fluctuates during episodes, tinnitus, and ear fullness. Some of the patients develop drop attacks called Tumarkin crisis, also known as otolithic crisis, and nausea [4, 5].

Meniere's disease or syndrome is one of the most common inner ear diseases. Its prevalence reported 3.5–513 per 100,000 in USA series [6]. It shows slightly female predominance 1.89:1 [7]. It is more common in white and older population; peak age is in the fourth and fifth decade but some early onset cases in children are reported [8, 9].

Meniere's usually starts in one ear, but bilateral disease is not uncommon. It may occur many years after the unilateral symptoms first started. Its prevalence is unclear and reported from 2 to 78% [9]. Familial Meniere's disease has been reported in 10–20% of cases [10]. Meniere's disease is strongly associated with Meniere's disease so as allergies.

 IntechOpen

Till this day, an effective treatment protocol is not established, because the pathogenesis of Meniere's disease is not clear.

2. Pathogenesis

Most common histopathologic finding is "endolymphatic hydrops" but the exact pathology is unknown. The Committee on Hearing and Equilibrium of American Academy of Otolaryngology Head and Neck Surgery's (AAO-HNS) definition of certain Meniere's disease contains histopathologial confirmation of endolymphatic hydrops [11].

Endolymph is produced by stria vascularis in the cochlea and by the dark cells in the vestibular labyrinth [12]. In autopsy studies, endolymphatic hydrops was observed in the temporal bones of patients who were diagnosed Meniere's disease, but not all individuals who had endolymphatic hydrops developed Meniere's disease symptoms [13, 14]. Perisaccular fibrosis and decreased endolymphatic duct size are observed in some of the patients. The CT images showed that individuals have hypoplastic endolymphatic sac and duct and inadequate periaqueductal pneumatization [15]. MRI studies showed that patients with Meniere's disease have significantly smaller and shorter drainage system [16]. After gadolinium enhancement, enhancement of endolymphatic sac and periventricular space was demonstrated in MRI [17, 18]. Nakashima et al. designed a study to demonstrate endolymphatic hydrops in Meniere's disease in 3 Tesla MRI. Gadolinium was injected transtympanically and MR images were taken a day after. They observed that the gadolinium moves first into the perilymphatic space and that can reveal the border between endolymph and perilymph. They successfully showed the endolymphatic hydrops in these patients [19]. Naganawa et al. study demonstrated same results with 1.5 Tesla MRI after intravenous administration of gadolinium. They reported their waiting time is much shorter (4 hours after contrast enhancement) and 95% success rate, while the intratympanic gadolinium method's rate of success is reported as 80–90% [20]. Imaging is also important as it helps in differential diagnosis of the other cases that could cause unilateral hearing loss, vertigo such as vestibular schwannoma.

It is hypothesized that the ruptures of membranous labyrinth and cicatrization in healing process could cause the drain blockage that leads to endolymphatic hydrops [21, 22]. Schuknect explained that, the ruptures of membranous labyrinth cause the leakage of potassium enriched endolymph to perilymph depolarize the nerve cells. Acute inactivation results with hearing loss and vertigo, after healing process of the chemical distribution of ions normalize; so the effects are reversible. Since the Meniere's disease takes its course through lifetime, the effects on the inner ear is irreversible at some point, so the hearing loss is permanent and vertigo attacks subdue [23]. However, this theory is not accepted by all; some authors suggested that ruptures are occurred rarely and not adequate to explain all the symptoms [24].

3. Etiology

Meniere's syndrome is the triad; fluctuating hearing loss, tinnitus, and episodes of vertigo; if the cause is unknown it is defined as Meniere's disease [25]. In experimental studies, the blockage of endolymphatic duct and its lead to endolymphatic hydrops is shown in animals. In order to create this, mechanical blockage, viral inoculation, and immune response-induced inflammation are used [26].

Some of the studies suggested that allergy and Meniere's disease could be linked. Derebery et al. studied patients who were diagnosed with Meniere's disease. The skin prick test results were positive of 41% of these patients, which were three times higher than general population [27]. Some mechanisms were proposed in order to explain the link between allergy and Meniere's disease.

1. The fenestrated blood vessels that are located in endolymphatic sac allow the antigen to enter that leads to mast cell degranulation. Inflammation around the perisaccular fibrous tissue and release of histamine cause vasodilatation and increase the secretion that causes endolymphatic sac resorption capacity over rules.

2. Immune complexes that enter the endolymphatic sac circulation through this fenestrated vessels start inflammation and increase vascular permeability.

3. Waldeyer's ring stimulated by viral antigens triggers T-cell migration to endolymphatic sac and leads to inflammation and excession of fluid production [28].

In order to demonstrate this relationship, Derebery et al. investigated the effects of allergen immunotherapy and elimination of food allergens in Meniere's disease patients. Their results were surprisingly positive. They reported that the improvement of symptoms of Meniere's disease and allergic symptoms were significant [29].

Another mechanism that is suggested is viral infection; however, no specific virus is identified [30].

Ischemia is another factor that is suggested in Meniere's disease mechanism [31]. Migraine and Meniere's disease link by vascular mechanism [32].

4. Diagnosis

In order to plan a treatment algorithm for Meniere's disease, it is important to diagnose it accurately. Diagnostic investigation is not bound to only one test result. The Committee on Hearing and Equilibrium of the AAO-HNS has described the symptoms. As per AAO-HNS, the major symptoms of Meniere's disease are vertigo, hearing loss, and tinnitus [11].

4.1 Vertigo

Spontaneous, rotational vertigo that last at least 20 minutes accompanied usually with nausea and vomiting which are the definitive spells of Meniere's disease. During the spell, horizontal or horizontal rotatory nystagmus is observed.

4.2 Hearing loss

Fluctuating hearing loss, commonly in low frequencies, is the most common audiological finding. In some cases, hearing loss is progressive and is usually unilateral.

Hearing loss is described as:

- the arithmetic mean of hearing thresholds of 250, 500, and 1000 Hz which is 15 dB or higher than the average of 1000, 2000, and 3000 Hz; or,

- average threshold of 500, 1000, 2000, and 3000 Hz which is 20 dB or higher in poorer ear in unilateral cases; or

- average threshold of 500, 1000, 2000, and 3000 Hz which is higher than 25 dB in bilateral cases.

About 10 dB change or more or 15% or more change in speech discrimination rate is considered clinically significant.

One of the prognostic factors that affects hearing function is duration of the disease [33]. It is documented by most of the authors [34–36]. Age is also an independent prognostic factor to determine hearing function and its responsiveness to medical treatment [37].

4.3 Tinnitus and aural fullness

It could be confirmed with the patients' history. Tinnitus is commonly of a low-frequency type [38]. Sometimes, patients describe it to be localized in affected ear or sense it in the whole head. Patients describe tinnitus differently from each other [39].

4.4 Clinical presentation

The initial symptom of Meniere's disease can be vertigo (37%), tinnitus (18%), fluctuating hearing loss (20%), or any combination of these. Only 25% of cases start with all of these symptoms [40].

Most of the patients describe recurrent vertigo attacks (96.2%) with tinnitus (91.1%) and ipsilateral hearing loss (87.7%) [41]. Most of the crippling symptom is vertigo. In an acute attack, it tends to stay 20 minutes to 24 hours [42].

The beginning of the Meniere's disease differs from patient to patient as well as the course of the disease. It is found that vertigo stops in 57% of the patients in 2 years and 71% of the cases in 8.3 years after the first onset [43].

Detailed clinical history should be taken as the first and most important step for diagnosis. Most of the distressing symptom is vertigo. It is usually present in horizontal axis, accompanied with nausea and vomiting. During this attack, horizontal or horizontal rotatory nystagmus could be observed.

Some of the patients could describe sudden drop attacks which were described by Tumarkin, and this symptom is named after him also called otolithic crisis of Tumarkin. This symptom is caused by utriculosaccular dysfunction [44]. Sudden changes in vertical gravity reference cause postural adjustments via vestibulospinal pathway and end up with sudden fall [45]. About 2–6% of patients with Meniere's disease were reported to experience drop attack [46].

Second common symptom is hearing loss usually accompanied with tinnitus and ear fullness sensation. Hearing loss is fluctuating, most in low frequencies and tends to be progressive; however, only 1–2% of patients end up with profound hearing loss [47]. Additionally, 43.6% of the patients have different perception of hearing between ears (diplacusis) and 56% recruitment [25].

Tinnitus description could be different between patients but it is usually nonpulsatile and could be continuous or appears only during the attack, or could get worse during the attacks.

The AAO-HNS Committee on Hearing and Equilibrium suggested staged diagnosis for Meniere's disease. They suggested to group patients in the order of their symptoms as possible, probable, definite, and certain Meniere's disease [11] (**Table 1**).

Possible Meniere's disease	• Episodic vertigo without documented hearing loss, or • Sensorineural hearing loss (fluctuating or flat) with disequilibrium but without definitive vertigo attacks
Probable Meniere's disease	• One definite vertigo episode • Documented hearing loss at least once • Tinnitus or ear fullness
Definite Meniere's disease	• Two or more definite vertigo attacks lasted at least 20 minutes • Documented hearing loss at least one • Tinnitus or ear fullness
Certain Meniere's disease	• Definite Meniere's disease • Histopathological confirmation of endolymphatic hydrops

Table 1.
Diagnosis of Meniere's disease.

Probable Meniere's disease	• Two or more spontaneous episodes of vertigo (each lasts 20 minutes to 24 hours) • Fluctuating aural symptoms on the affected ear (tinnitus, hearing loss, or aural fullness) • Other vestibular diseases were excluded
Definite Meniere's disease	• Two or more spontaneous episodes of vertigo (each lasts 20 minutes to 12 hours) • Low- to mid-frequency sensorineural hearing loss in affected ear (documented with audiometry) at least on one occasion (before, during, or after the vertigo episode) • Fluctuating aural symptoms on the affected ear (tinnitus, hearing loss, or aural fullness) • Other vestibular diseases were excluded

Table 2.
Amended 2015 criteria for diagnosis of Meniere's disease.

The AAO-HNS Committee on Hearing and Equilibrium revised their diagnostic criteria in 2015. The new definition of "Definite" and "Probable" Meniere's disease is summed up in **Table 2** [48].

4.4.1 Diagnostic workup

To treat Meniere's disease successfully, diagnosis should be confirmed. There is not a single test exists to confirm Meniere's disease alone, so the patient should be evaluated with possible diagnostic tests.

4.4.2 Videonystagmography

Eye movements are observed after caloric or vestibular stimulation. Caloric response is found to decrease in 48–73.5% of the patients' affected ear, and complete absence is reported in 6–11% of patients [49, 50].

4.4.3 Electrocochleography

Summation potentials are larger and more negative in Meniere's disease. Most valuable ratio is summation potential/action potential. SP/AP ratio is found to be increased in Meniere's disease. However, this is not definitive, and only 62% of patients with Meniere's disease have elevated ratios [51].

4.4.4 Dehydrating agents

Dehydrating agent such as glycerol, urea used to reduce endolymph volume and improvement of symptoms were such as improved hearing, reduction of SP negativity in electrocochleography, trying to be observed. It is reported 60% sensitivity for Meniere's disease [52].

4.4.5 Vestibular evoked myopotentials

Loud clicks are used to stimulate stapedial movement in order to stimulate the saccule. Stimulation saccule triggers the pathway that relaxes sternocleidomastoid muscle. Normal ear response is recorded as 500 Hz, and affected ear's response is recorded in elevated thresholds with flattened tuning [53].

The AAO-HNS's guideline is suggested in 1995 and does not contain these diagnostic vestibular battery; it is only suggested to the use of full audiometric workup.

One of the recent guidelines for diagnosis and treatment of Meniere's disease is from French Otorhinolaryngology-Head and Neck Surgery Society (SFORL) in 2016. They describe that "definite" Meniere's disease could be diagnosed if another cause could not be described to explain the following four clinical findings;

- two or more rotational vertigo attacks that last 2 minutes to 12 hours or, Tumarkin's crises;
- low-frequency hearing loss on two consecutive frequencies, 30 dB or more if the other ear hearing is normal, or 35 dB or more if hearing is affected bilaterally; and
- tinnitus or aural fullness; and
- fluctuating otologic findings.

MRI of inner ear is suggested to rule out cerebellopontine angle or endolymphatic sac tumors, anatomic deformity, or a degenerative pathology such as multiple sclerosis that could mimic the symptoms of Meniere's disease. Also audiovestibular workup could lead the clinician to intralabyrintine pressure disorder. The workup should include at least pure-tone and speech audiometry with VNG or VEMP or VHIT [54].

5. Treatment

Ideal treatment should stop vertigo attacks, restore hearing, and get rid of tinnitus and ear fullness. Unfortunately, ideal treatment is absent nowadays. Our limited knowledge of pathophysiology of the disease makes it impossible to treat patients ideally. Also symptoms and course of the disease differ between patients, so treatment should be individualized.

The aim of the treatment is to reduce frequency and severity of vertigo attacks and improve hearing results [55]. All current treatment options are symptomatic.

Due to natural course of the disease, vertigo attacks of 60–80% of patients improve without any intervention [56, 57]. Patients who refused to take any medical or surgical assistance had spontaneous improvement of their symptoms at the rate of 71% [43]. Green et al. reported complete vertigo control in 50% of the patients, partial control in 28% of the patients, and only 17% of their patient needed medical treatment in their 14 years of follow-up [58].

Treatment options are decided upon the remaining hearing, severity, and intensity of vertigo attacks. Meniere's disease is progressive on hearing levels of the patient; some of them develop profound hearing loss which also could affect the other ear. In order to plan a treatment scheme for a patient, these conditions should be assessed. It has destructive and progressive nature, so the first step of treatment should contain more conservative treatment options. If symptom control could not be obtained, destructive treatment options should be considered.

AAO-HNS suggested a staging system based on a four-tone average of 500, 1000, 2000, and 3000 Hz on the worst pure-tone audiometry, and this system should be obtained to the patients who were diagnosed with "definite" or "certain" Meniere's disease (**Table 3**) [11].

International Consensus (ICON) on treatment of the Meniere's disease proposed a treatment algorithm in 2018 (**Figure 1**) [59].

ICON's proposal for treatment algorithm summarizes the logic of the treatment for Meniere's disease. When the course of the disease is considered, Meniere's disease could make the affected ear to deteriorate and also could affect the other ear

Stage	Four-tone average (dB)
I	25 or less
II	26–40
III	41–70
IV	>70

Table 3.
Staging of definite and certain Meniere's disease.

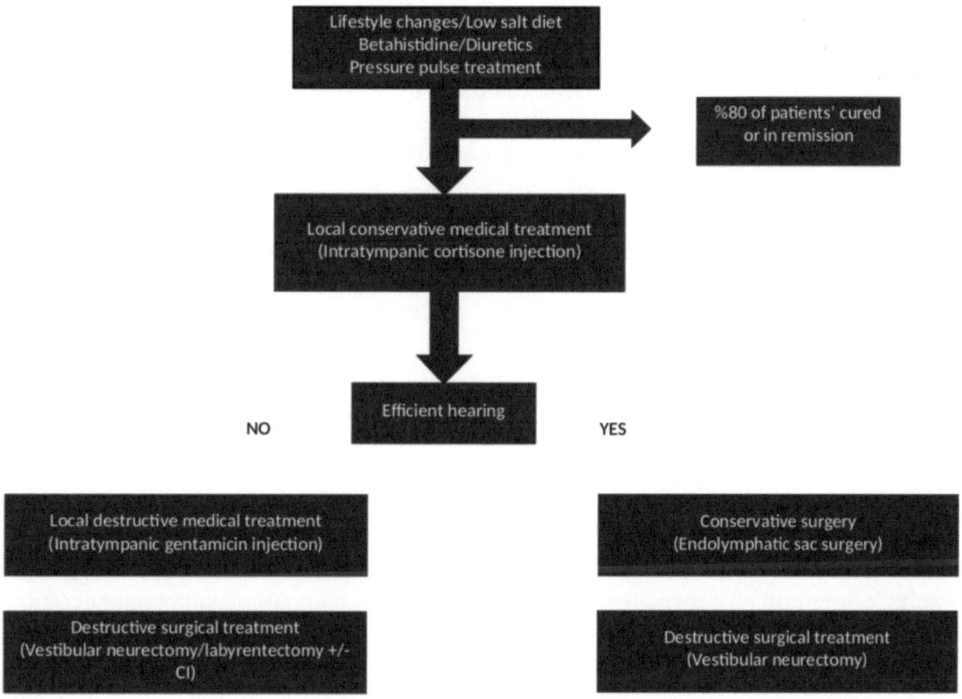

Figure 1.
Treatment algorithm of Meniere's disease proposed by ICON in 2018.

at any time. Most logical approach for treatment is starting with less invasive option and assessing the patient periodically. If the suggested treatment fails, more invasive methods should be offered.

Also in SFORL guideline of treatment, a step-by-step approach from conservative to destructive is suggested.

If a patient seeks for medical attention during vertigo attack, treatment is symptomatic. The rest of the chapter contains nonsurgical treatment options, acute attack treatment, and vestibular rehabilitation options.

5.1 Preventive treatment options

5.1.1 Lifestyle changes and low salt diet

The first line of treatment is to encourage the patient to change his lifestyle into a healthier one. Regulation of sleeping cycle, avoiding stress, caffeine, alcohol, and tobacco, and changing into a low salt diet should be advised [60–62]. Caffeine is accused to increase the endolymph volume due to its sympathomimetic actions, and it is suggested to be restricted to 100 mg/day by AAO-HNS [63]. More active lifestyle should be offered, like taking at least 20 minutes of walking.

Low salt diet has been suggested to Meniere's disease patients since the 1930s, where daily intake of sodium is recommended to be under 2 grams [64, 65]. Low salt intake increases serum aldosterone levels [66]. It has been found that endolymphatic sac contains receptors for mineral corticoids [67]. Aldosterone controls Na/K ATPase, thiazide-sensitive Na/Cl co-transporter, and epithelial Na channels which are also expressed on endolymphatic sac [68–73]. It has been shown that canrenoate, an aldosterone antagonist, reduced electrical potentials of endolymphatic sac after applied [74, 75]. Elevation of aldosterone levels may increase the endolymph absorption [70]. However, restriction of salt intake could not be proven to change the levels of sodium of plasma and endolymph [64, 65, 76].

In Miyashita et al.'s study, Meniere's disease patients were grouped in order to their sodium intake. After initiation of low sodium diet, patients were observed for 2 years. Low sodium group (daily intake of 3 grams or less) had better hearing levels and less vertigo attacks than high sodium group (daily intake more than 3 grams). However, serum aldosterone levels were not different although low sodium group had higher serum levels [77].

Also Tadros and colleagues investigated elder population and those who had higher serum aldosterone levels had better hearing levels, and they suggested that aldosterone might have a protective effect on hearing [78].

Low sodium intake has known benefits on cardiovascular health; hence, there is no harm to suggest it.

5.1.2 Betahistine

Betahistine is a weak histamine H1 receptor agonist and a potent histamine H3 receptor antagonist.

It is suggested to improve microvascular circulation in stria vascularis that reduces the endolymph pressure [79], and it inhibits vestibular nuclei activity that results longer and easier recovery [80, 81]. It reaches its peak plasma concentration in 1 hour, and maximal therapeutic effects start in 3–4 hours after intake [82].

Betahistine is a popular agent in Europe and Japan. FDA does not approve its use in vertigo as it is not commonly used in the USA. Its beneficial effects are based on the clinical observation; some studies report favorable results on vertigo control and hearing improvement and some studies do not. In betahistine's case, literature findings are controversial. In SFORL guideline, betahistine is suggested as the first line of treatment.

Tootoonchi et al. reported improvement of 6.35 dB in hearing levels after 6 months of betahistine administration [37]. However, patient's first hearing levels should be considered; if the patient has poor hearing levels at the first visit, he is less likely to benefit from the treatment [36]. Cochrane reviews support the positive effect of betahistine on vertigo attack frequency and hearing levels. They highlighted the fact that the investigated studies have serious study design flaws and tend to bias [83]. Therapeutic benefits of betahistine were reported in Nauta's meta-analysis [84].

BEMED study is a multi-central, placebo-controlled study that investigates the effects of betahistine. The results on vestibular symptoms were not any different compared to placebo [85]. In order to establish the benefits of betahistine, more well-designed, placebo-controlled studies are required.

Literature seems to be controversial but it is suggested as the first line of treatment in the European, French, and Japanese guidelines as its beneficial effects on patients are observed clinically.

5.1.3 Diuretics

Another treatment agent widely used for Meniere's disease treatment is diuretics. Thiazide group of diuretics is usually suggested. The cells that produce endolymph, such as dark cells and stria vascularis, contain carbonic anhydrase. Carbonic anhydrase inhibitors like acetazolamide are recommended in order to reduce the production endolymph [86].

Recent systematic review on diuretics was conducted by Crowson and colleagues. They reviewed four retrospective studies. One of the studies compared betahistine and diuretics and reported improved results on vertigo in both groups but lack of placebo group [87]. In another study, diuretics showed beneficial effects on vestibular symptoms compared to placebo [88]. Another placebo-controlled retrospective study reported beneficial effects of hydrochlorothiazide on hearing loss and vertigo control [89]. Most of the studies have low level of evidence. Cochrane report in 2006 on diuretics reported beneficial but it highlighted the fact that most of the studies were lack of high quality of evidence [90]. However, studies indicate improvement in vertigo and lesser effect on hearing. Still they are suggested as the first line of treatment options in many guidelines.

5.1.4 Pulse pressure treatment

Around three decades ago, it has been reported that positive pressure to middle ear could have helped release of Meniere's disease's symptoms [91]. The underlying mechanism is still unclear. Meniett device was introduced by Medtronic company in 2000 and approved by FDA for Meniere's disease treatment. After insertion of a ventilation tube, the device is placed to external ear canal and sends low-pressure pulses.

There are many studies about Meniett's effect on Meniere's disease and symptom control. Gates et al.'s randomized controlled studies showed benefits of Meniett device in short term. They demonstrated a significant decrease of vertigo attacks in first 3 months but this could not be observed in long term [92]. Other studies reached different conclusions about Meniett.

Ahsan et al. suggested that Meniett could be useful for Meniere's disease treatment, but Syed and van Sonsbeek were unable to show this effect in their randomized controlled studies where they compared the device effect to placebo [93–95].

Recent meta-analysis reported that Meniett device provided complete remission of 52% of patients and 34% of patients had not complete but significant release of symptoms [96]. This meta-analysis also investigated the suggested treatment protocols. Initiation of Meniett after 2 weeks of ventilation tube insertion seemed to have better control over the symptoms. Effects on vertigo seem to begin in first 6 months, reach its peak in 6–18 months, and stabilize after 18 months. Also it was observed that the shorter initiation of the therapy after placement of ventilation tube had a better effect on hearing preservation and vertigo control [96].

However, some authors have different opinions when it comes to ventilation tubes. They suggest that ventilation tube insertion alone could control Meniere's disease symptoms [97–100]. In hypoxia theory, it is hypothesized that vertigo attacks are triggered by anoxia in inner ear, which can decrease endolymphatic potentials and microcirculation of cochlea [101, 102]. Ventilation tube enriches middle ear oxygenation and helps anoxic environment of inner ear [103]. Also ventilation tube decreases the middle ear pressure, and it is hypothesized that this could help to balance the increased inner ear pressure that could lead to Meniere's attack [104]. It remains inconclusive that the decrease of symptoms after Meniett device is only from the ventilation tube or ventilation tube insertion alone. However, Zhang et al.'s meta-analysis reviewed studies that compare Meniett to placebo device and reached a conclusion. They report that if the interval between ventilation tube insertion and Meniett device is longer than 2 weeks, beneficial effects may be due to Meniett device alone [96].

Recent Cochrane database reviewed Meniett device-based studies that were published until 2014. Randomized controlled trials that compare Meniett and placebo devices were included in their study. Due to heterogeneity of data, calculation of outcome was reported not possible. Most of the studies found no significant difference between Meniett and placebo on vertigo control. Only one study showed a significant vertigo control after 8 weeks of usage of Meniett. Secondary outcomes like improvement on hearing, Meniett group significantly had better outcomes with 7.38 dB increase, effects on tinnitus and aural fullness could not be determined due to heterogeneity of data. Their conclusion is that data due to these studies are not adequate to determine the beneficial effects of Meniett [95].

Long-term results of Meniett device was published by Dornhoffer et al. Treated patients' improvement rates reported 75%, similar of untreated patients [105]. University of Colorado stated that the device is expensive and lacks cost-beneficiality [106].

None of the studies that investigated Meniett device reported any complications. Therefore it is harmless to propose this treatment. It is advised as the first-line treatment of ICON's guideline as well as Italian and Australian treatment algorithms [59, 95]. It is reported as the most common second-line treatment option in the USA [107]. With its potential benefits and low risk of complication rates, Meniett device could be advised to patients.

5.1.5 Ventilation tubes

Though it is a surgical procedure, it is minimally invasive so its effects on Meniere's disease will be discussed in this chapter. After myringotomy of the anteroinferior quadrant of tympanic membrane, ventilation tube could be inserted as an office procedure. Sugawara et al. and Montandon et al. reported that ventilation tube insertion has control over Meniere's disease symptoms without further treatment [97, 98].

Kimura and Hutta's experimental study on guinea pigs is that the middle ear ventilation reduced endolymphatic hydrops. It is hypothesized that ventilation of middle ear decreases the pressure in middle and inner ear [103].

Tumarkin was the first physician who introduced ventilation tubes as a treatment option in 1966. Tumarkin also reported that eustachian tube dysfunction is correlated with endolymphatic hydrops and his data was supported by Lall [108, 109]. However, Cinnamond, Hall, and Brackmann reported that eustachian tube dysfunction was not always observed with Meniere's disease patients and insertion of ventilation tube could worsen the symptoms of patients [110, 111].

Montadon et al. reported that complete remission or improvement rates of their patients were 82%. They also reported that the patient whose ventilation tube blocked had recurrence of symptoms and immediate relief after reinsertion of ventilation tubes [98]. Thomsen published results of patients who received transmastoid endolymphatic decompression surgery compared with patients who were inserted ventilation tube. Each group had significant control over their symptoms but found no difference between these groups [112].

Among the most recent studies in literature in 2015, Ogawa et al. studied ventilation tube insertion and its effects on intractable Meniere's disease patients. All of their patients were treated medically at least 6 months before ventilation tube insertion was advised. After a year, 20% of their patients had complete remission, 47% had partial remission. Two years later, complete vertigo control rates increased to 47%. Secondary benefits of procedure on hearing levels had no significant difference. They reported that ventilation tube insertion could be beneficial and postponed more invasive procedures [100]. Therefore, it could be advised as a first-line surgical procedure to patients who have symptoms after medical treatment.

The SFORL guideline does not recommend this procedure due to lack of evidence [54]. Not considered in ICON's guideline or the European Position Statement on diagnosis and Treatment of Meniere's disease [59, 113].

However, it is worthwhile to try because literature findings of some authors showed beneficial effects and it is minimally invasive and has low-complication rates.

5.1.6 Intratympanic steroid injections

Intratympanic steroid treatment will be discussed in later chapters.

5.2 Treatment of acute attacks

It is important to control the effects and related vegetative symptoms of vertigo during acute attack. Meniere's attacks are sudden onset and could last 20 minutes to 24 hours. In order to suppress the symptoms, benzodiazepines, meclizine, or other antihistamines could be used [106]. Drugs that are used to suppress the symptoms of Meniere's disease have no effect on progression of the disease.

Antihistamines, such as dimenhidrate, meclizine, benzodiazepines, and scopolamine, and anti-dopamines, which had antiemetic effects, such as metoclopramide and fenotiazines, are used to suppress the vestibular symptoms. These agents also have sedative effects that could help to reduce the patients' anxiety. Diazepam is effective on GABA receptors in vestibular nucleus and inhibits their response. It should only be used during acute attack because the long-term usage decreases vestibular compensation mechanisms. Dimenhidrate could also provide relief during acute attack but it could affect concentration and cause dizziness in long term [114].

Diazepam inhibits vestibular response with its effect on GABA-ergic receptors located in cerebellar system [115]. However, clinical and experimental studies show that the long-term usage of diazepam prolongs the vestibular compensation [116, 117].

Meclizine is useful to reduce vegetative symptoms like nausea, benzodiazepines are also well tolerated anxiolytic, in order of intractable vomiting promethazine suppositories could be used [106].

Transdermal scopolamine patches reaches therapeutic blood level 4 hours after placement and release drug to system 72 hours; however, this could not be useful because of the attacks' sudden onset nature [118].

Intravenous lidocaine has found to be effective during acute attack of Meniere's disease [119].

5.3 Vestibular rehabilitation and psychological support

Meniere's disease is a chronic attack characterized by their sudden onset. It is observed by most of the physicians that it also burdens patients psychologically. Also it is observed that stress and anxiety could trigger the attacks. Increase of vertigo severity is associated with worse quality of life scores of Meniere's disease [120]. Most of the guidelines suggest psychological support and behavioral therapy for the patients so they could have a better understanding of their condition and help themselves to cooperate with this condition.

Van Cruijsen et al. suggested that the symptoms could be worsened in negative emotional state [121]. Many studies reported the relation between symptoms and behavioral characteristics; the worse perception of the disease could create a vicious circle [122–124]. Patients suffering from Meniere's disease were found to be having more stress-causative behavioral characteristics than normal controls. This information leads to hypothesis that higher stress-related hormone levels could cause endolymphatic hydrops [124]. Another study by Van Cruijsen that assesses the psychological state of Meniere's disease patients compared to patients who had chronic vestibular diseases documented that 63% of Meniere's disease patients had psychologic pathology, such as depression or anxiety, but found no significant difference between non-Meniere's disease patients. It is also reported that Meniere's disease patients quality of life questionnaire results were worse than normal results [125].

Yokota et al. studied the treatment outcomes of both surgical and nonsurgical treatment due to patients' psychological status. Patients who had no mental distress had benefitted from both of the treatments more than the patients who had mental problems. Also surgical treatment options tend to have been found more beneficial over nonsurgical treatment among the patients who had psychological disorders. In order to improve treatment results of both surgical and nonsurgical options, it is advised that psychological support is necessary [126].

Better understanding of the disease and psychological state and their relation with better results seem to be beneficial for patients. Healthier psychology, encouragement to participate in active life, and providing psychological support in any chronic illness are important to help patients to remain as functional individuals in the society.

Traditionally, vestibular rehabilitation is ineffective in episodic vertigo patients. Stable conditions are better candidates for successful rehabilitation. Due to its chronic and progressive nature, rehabilitation of these patients is tricky. In order to obtain rehabilitation, physical therapy must be customized. It is not advised to initiate a rehabilitation program in acute onset.

The success of rehabilitation depends on the patient. First step of a successful rehabilitation program is education of the patient. Each patient is unique, and their characteristics, mental status, and understanding capacity differ between each other. Patients have to be informed about their disease, its nature and treatment options. Detailed explanation should be given about the effectiveness of physical therapy, coping mechanisms, and possible sequels for each person's understanding level. It is also important to correct the patient if they were misinformed [127].

Before customizing a rehabilitation program, the patient should be examined systemically. Mecagni et al.'s study demonstrated that limited ankle motion range affects the patient's performance on balance tests [127]. Lower extremities should be examined on their functional levels and sense of proprioception. Impaired vision could affect oculomotor functions negatively. In order to determine relationships between the input mechanisms of balance system, posturography could be used if it is available [128]. It is reported that static platform posturography is more sensitive and specific in Meniere's disease than caloric and rotational tests, both in diagnosing and detecting other deficits that accompany these patients' vestibular system [129, 130].

Although there is not a test battery that could predict the effects of attacks on patients daily life, most of the patients describe the attacks debilitating [131]. Most of the time attacks occur suddenly and being prepared for those attacks is important. It should be discussed with the patient about special sensations or feelings before the attack. At least half of the patients could identify a trigger [132]. In order to identify these conditions, a symptom diary could be advised.

Some protective advices should be given to the patient to be performed during the attack. Also most of the patients tend to close their eyes during the attack, and it should be taught that keeping their eyes open and targeting them onto something would help them to suppress nystagmus [127]. Instead of panicking over symptoms, they should be advised to stay calm and sit or lie down in order to prevent themselves from further injuries.

When the attack subdued, refractory effects could continue to debilitate the patient. The patient should be advised to avoid any sudden movements. In order to minimize the effects on their personal lifestyles, some modifications should be advised like performing daily activities, sitting instead of standing while cooking, dressing up, etc.

In order to prevent patients' social isolation, patients should be encouraged about informing their social circle about their condition. Also series of exercises should be programmed for each patient's current status, and patients should be encouraged to participate in social life. In our clinic, we advise our patients to go to a mall for window shopping. It helps patients to overcome their fear to be in public, helps them to use visual object to train their vestibulo-ocular system, and also improves their walking and sense of proprioception. In addition to these advises, if a specific problem was found on their posturography, it is consulted with related departments.

Rehabilitation and its importance are well documented in Meniere's disease patients who received a destructive protocol [133–135]. However, studies about the effects of vestibular rehabilitation on patients who suffer from post-vertigo disequilibrium are limited. Clendaniel and Tucci reported the importance of vestibular rehabilitation of patients after vertigo attack [136].

Gottshall et al.'s study demonstrated the beneficial effects of vestibular exercises on post-vertigo symptoms with unilateral Meniere's disease. Patients reported that their balance function was significantly improved, only experiencing subtle discomfort [137]. In bilateral disease, it is reported by Cohen et al. that vestibular rehabilitation was not effective and advised to evaluate other adaptive strategies with these patients [138].

Vestibular rehabilitation between attacks could help patients to cooperate with disease and help them to keep their functionality levels up. Vestibular rehabilitation's effect on patients' mental status is not reported in the current literature but logically it could improve mental health. Recent guidelines recommend behavioral therapies and vestibular rehabilitation programs.

5.4 Hearing loss and tinnitus in Meniere's disease

Meniere's disease symptoms are episodic vertigo attacks, fluctuating hearing loss, tinnitus, and ear fullness. Most disturbing symptom of this condition is vertigo according to most of the studies that evaluated the quality of life scores of the patients. So the preservation of hearing function and reducing the tinnitus intensity are always evaluated as secondary outcomes in studies. During follow-up of the patients, it is important to document hearing levels because remained hearing function is the key factor in decision-making process of the treatment.

One of the diagnostic criteria of Meniere's disease according to AAO-HNS's guideline is hearing loss.

It is recommended to stage the disease and underline as an important factor to monitor the treatment results [11].

In ICON's guideline, destructive treatment options are recommended if there is no functional hearing left [59]. Hearing loss is usually located in lower frequencies, and in early stages of the disease, it has a fluctuating pattern [139, 140]. In later phases, it could decrease, and after 5–10 years, hearing thresholds usually settle to 50–60 dB as well as speech discrimination scores decrease to 50–60% [141]. Tinnitus is mostly a low-frequency type due to hearing loss, which could be localized to affected ear and could be described globally [38]. Low-frequency tinnitus is difficult to be masked with environmental sounds [142].

Havia et al. reported the relationship between vertigo, hearing loss, and tinnitus. Patients with more profound hearing loss had worse outcomes on their posturography tests and caloric test responses found decreased on the affected ear [35]. Recent studies demonstrated that hearing loss in these patients is associated with sensory element degeneration [143].

The intensity of tinnitus reported to increase with duration symptoms. Intense tinnitus is found to be related with hearing loss specifically at 500 Hz. However, vertigo attack frequency or duration of the attacks was not related with tinnitus intensity [35]. Gentamicin injections proven to be effective to reduce the tinnitus but surgical interventions found to be ineffective on tinnitus control [144, 145]. In order to compensate with tinnitus, behavioral therapy should be advised. Betahistine and nasal oxytocin were studied in Meniere's disease and they reported to decrease tinnitus perception but data are limited [146, 147]. Cochlear implants have reported that they decrease tinnitus significantly; although the data are limited and still relatively new, it is reported to decrease tinnitus of patients after 6 months [148].

5.5 Treatment of bilateral Meniere's disease

Bilateral Meniere's disease prevalence is reported in 2–47% of the cases, and it could occur after several years of the first onset of the disease [9]. Temporal bone studies suggest that bilateral Meniere's disease incidence is higher and bilateral endolymphatic hydrops observed 25–30% of the inspected temporal bones [149–151]. Bilateral Meniere's disease should be treated conservatively; bilateralization could occur at any time, and there is no test that could prevent this. This condition is the main reason of the emphasis on being conservative while choosing the treatment option.

Meniere's disease rarely start bilaterally, it usually starts with unilaterally [152–154]. Most of the cases, contralateral involvement occurs after 2–5 years after the first initiation of symptoms [155]. Clinical presentation of these cases is different from each other. Most important step in diagnosis is suspicion and knowledge of the possible nature of the disease could affect the contralateral side at some point of patients' follow-up. Severity of the disease should be established independently for each ear, in pure-tone audiometry average of 500, 1000, 2000, and 3000 Hz >25 dB [11]. Tinnitus is reported to be more intense in bilateral Meniere's patients. Also they reported that patients who had bilateral Meniere's disease had significantly longer history of disease and worse pure-tone average [35].

In EcoG, Iseli and Gibson reported that summation potential/action potential ratio has a limited value to determine endolymphatic hydrops and should be combined with summation potential amplitude ans summating potential bias ratio [156]. Lin et al. proposed to combine VEMP tuning and VEMP thresholds to detect the hydrops in the contralateral ear before the symptoms' onset [157]. In imaging, studies suggest that affected side has endolymphatic dilatation and due to this perilymph volume seem decreased [158]. Combination of these diagnostic strategies could help physicians to detect bilateral involvement and avoid from destructive procedures in suspected patients.

In ICON's guideline, they reported that the bilateral tendency of the disease attributed as an important factor of most clinic treatment protocol shift from intratympanic gentamicin to intratympanic steroid. Also as a surgical treatment option, endolymphatic sac procedures are recommended for bilateral Meniere's disease [59]. In SFORL guideline, gentamicin injections are contraindicated in single intact ear or bilateral Meniere's disease. They recommend endolymphatic sac surgery if medical treatments failed in bilateral Meniere's disease. Destructive surgeries such as vestibular neurectomy and labyrinthectomy are not recommended in bilateral Meniere's disease [54].

Treatment options of bilateral disease are restricted. Conservative treatment options should be advised and symptomatic treatment should be prescribed during attack. Peterson et al. conduct a survey study among American otorhinolaryngologists about their choice of treatment with patient who had only hearing ear and most common option is Meniett device when other conservative treatment options failed. After Meniett, intratympanic steroid injection comes second in their choice of treatment. Endolymphatic sac procedures come in third; first decompression is advised than shunt procedures. Selective vestibular nerve section comes later [107].

Intratympanic steroid injection could be advised to patients with bilateral Meniere's disease. Recent randomized controlled study conducted in 2005 reported that intratympanic steroid injections are the effective way of treatment [159]. However, another study found no difference between intratympanic steroid injection and saline injection [160, 161]. The literature findings are controversial.

Intravenous streptomycin sulfate in debilitating bilateral Meniere's disease reported to reduce the symptoms [162–164]. If complete or near complete bilateral hypo-function has occurred, streptomycin sulfate is found to be effective [163]. Immune-mediated bilateral Meniere's disease is a subgroup of Meniere's disease, and methotrexate treatment is found to be effective on symptom control [165]. Another treatment option for immune-mediated group is systemic steroids, its efficacy is reported in a few studies [153, 166–170]. Prospective study on treatment of bilateral Meniere's disease with systemic steroids reported significant improvement on decrease in vertigo attacks but had no effect on hearing loss or tinnitus or aural fullness [170].

Surgical option of these patients is endolymphatic sac surgery; it has lowest complication rates on sensorineural hearing loss, <2% [171]. Kitahara et al.'s study reported the results of patients who had endolymphatic sac drainage with and without insertion of steroid induced silastic and nonsurgical group. The vertigo control rates were similar in surgery groups with or without steroid, but hearing levels of steroid group had better long-term results than nonsteroid surgery group and nonsurgical group [172]. Their findings were also supported with review of Wetmore. In order of retractable disease ablative surgeries combined with cochlear implant insertion should be considered.

Author details

Yetkin Zeki Yilmaz*, Begum Bahar Yilmaz and Aysegul Batioglu-Karaaltın
Istanbul University-Cerrahpasa Medical Faculty ENT, Istanbul, Turkey

*Address all correspondence to: dr_yzy@hotmail.com

References

[1] Pearce JMS. Marie-Jean-Pierre Flourens (1794-1867) and cortical localization. European Neurology. 2009; **61**(5):311-314. DOI: 10.1159/000206858

[2] Baloh RW. Prosper Ménière and his disease. Archives of Neurology. 2001. DOI: 10.1001/archneur.58.7.1151

[3] Knapp HJ. A Clinical Analysis of the Inflammatory Affections of the Inner Ear.; 1871

[4] Perez-Fernandez N, Montes-Jovellar L, Cervera-Paz J, Domenech-Vadillo E. Auditory and vestibular assessment of patients with Ménière's disease who suffer Tumarkin attacks. Audiology and Neurotology. 2010. DOI: 10.1159/000310899

[5] Hägnebo C, Andersson G, Melin L. Correlates of vertigo attacks in Meniere's disease. Psychotherapy and Psychosomatics. 1998. DOI: 10.1159/000012296

[6] Alexander TH, Harris JP. Current epidemiology of Meniere's syndrome. Otolaryngologic Clinics of North America. 2010. DOI: 10.1016/j.otc.2010.05.001

[7] Shojaku H, Watanabe Y, Fujisaka M, et al. Epidemiologic characteristics of definite Ménière's disease in Japan: A long-term survey of Toyama and Niigata prefectures. ORL; Journal for Oto-rhino-laryngology and its Related Specialties. 2005. DOI: 10.1159/000089413

[8] Choung YH, Park K, Kim CH, Kim HJ, Kim K. Rare cases of Ménière's disease in children. The Journal of Laryngology and Otology. 2006. DOI: 10.1017/S0022215106000569

[9] House JW, Doherty JK, Fisher LM, Derebery MJ, Berliner KI. Meniere's disease: Prevalence of contralateral ear involvement. Otology & Neurotology. 2006. DOI: 10.1097/00129492-200604000-00011

[10] Morrison AW, Mowbray JF, Williamson R, Sheeka S, Sodha N, Koskinen N. On genetic and environmental factors in Menière's disease. The American Journal of Otology. 1994

[11] Committee on Hearing and Equilibrium. Committee on hearing and equilibrium guidelines for the diagnosis and evaluation of therapy in Meniere's disease. Otolaryngology–Head and Neck Surgery. 1995;**113**(3):181-185. DOI: 10.1016/S0194-5998(95)70102-8

[12] Jansson B, Rask-Andersen H. Erythrocyte removal and blood clearance in the endolymphatic sac. An experimental and TEM study. Acta Oto-Laryngologica. 1996

[13] Rauch SD, Merchant SN, Thedinger BA. Meniere's syndrome and endolymphatic hydrops: Double-blind temporal bone study. The Annals of Otology, Rhinology, and Laryngology. 1989. DOI: 10.1177/000348948909801108

[14] Wackym PA. Histopathologic findings in Meniere's disease. Otolaryngology and Head and Neck Surgery. 1995. DOI: 10.1016/S0194-5998(95)70307-1

[15] Valvassori GE, Dobben GD. Multidirectional and computerized tomography of the vestibular aqueduct in Meniere's disease. The Annals of Otology, Rhinology, and Laryngology. 1984. DOI: 10.1177/000348948409300604

[16] Albers FWJ, Van Weissenbruch R, Casselman JW. 3DFT-magnetic resonance imaging of the inner ear in Meniere's disease. Acta

Oto-Laryngologica. 1994. DOI: 10.3109/00016489409126111

[17] Fitzgerald DC, Mark AS. Endolymphatic duct/sac enhancement on gadolinium magnetic resonance imaging of the inner ear: Preliminary observations and case reports. The American Journal of Otology. 1996

[18] Carfrae MJ, Holtzman A, Eames F, Parnes SM, Lupinetti A. 3 Tesla delayed contrast magnetic resonance imaging evaluation of Meniere's disease. The Laryngoscope. 2008. DOI: 10.1097/MLG.0b013e31815c1a61

[19] Nakashima T, Naganawa S, Sugiura M, et al. Visualization of endolymphatic hydrops in patients with Meniere's disease. The Laryngoscope. 2007;**117**(3):415-420. DOI: 10.1097/MLG.0b013e31802c300c

[20] Naganawa S, Nakashima T. Visualization of endolymphatic hydrops with MR imaging in patients with Ménière's disease and related pathologies: Current status of its methods and clinical significance. Japanese Journal of Radiology. 2014; **32**(4):191-204. DOI: 10.1007/s11604-014-0290-4

[21] Schuknecht HFIM. Pathophysiology of Meniere's disease. In: Pfaltz CR, editor. Controversial Aspects of Meniere's Disease. New York: Georg Thieme; 1986

[22] Flock Å, Flock B. Micro-lesions in Reissner's membrane evoked by acute hydrops. Audiology & Neuro-Otology. 2003. DOI: 10.1159/000069002

[23] Schuknecht HF. The pathophysiology of Meniere's disease. The American Journal of Otology;**5**(6): 526-527

[24] Brown DH, McClure JA, Downar-Zapolski Z. The membrane rupture theory of Menière's disease–is it valid? The Laryngoscope. 1988. DOI: 10.1288/00005537-198806000-00003

[25] Paparella MM. Pathogenesis of Meniere's disease and Meniere's syndrome. Acta Oto-Laryngologica. 1983. DOI: 10.3109/00016488309122996

[26] Kimura RS. Animal models of inner ear vascular disturbances. American Journal of Otolaryngology - Head and Neck Medicine and Surgery. 1986. DOI: 10.1016/S0196-0709(86)80042-4

[27] Derebery MJ, Berliner KI. Prevalence of allergy in Meniere's disease. Otolaryngology-Head and Neck Surgery. 2000. DOI: 10.1016/S0194-5998(99)80287-3

[28] Derebery MJ, Berliner KI. Allergy and its relation to Meniere's disease. Otolaryngologic Clinics of North America. 2010. DOI: 10.1016/j.otc.2010.05.004

[29] Derebery MJ. Allergic management of Meniere's disease: An outcome study. Otolaryngology-Head and Neck Surgery. 2000. DOI: 10.1016/S0194-5998(00)70235-X

[30] Bergström T, Edström S, Tjellström A, Vahlne A. Ménière's disease and antibody reactivity to herpes simplex virus type 1 polypeptides. American Journal of Otolaryngology and Head and Neck Surgery. 1992. DOI: 10.1016/0196-0709(92)90051-T

[31] Lee KS, Kimura RS. Ischemia of the endolymphatic sac. Acta Oto-Laryngologica. 1992. DOI: 10.3109/00016489209137456

[32] Radtke A, Lempert T, Gresty MA, Brookes GB, Bronstein AM, Neuhauser H. Migraine and Ménière's disease: Is there a link? Neurology. 2002. DOI: 10.1212/01.WNL.0000036903.22461.39

[33] Paparella MM, Mcdermott JC, Sousa LCA. Meniere's disease and the peak audiogram. Archives of Otolaryngology. 1982. DOI: 10.1001/archotol.1982.00790570021005

[34] Katsarkas A. Hearing loss and vestibular dysfunction in Meniere's disease. Acta Oto-Laryngologica. 1996. DOI: 10.3109/00016489609137819

[35] Havia M, Kentala E, Pyykkö I. Hearing loss and tinnitus in Meniere's disease. Auris, Nasus, Larynx. 2002; **29**(2):115-119. DOI: 10.1016/S0385-8146(01)00142-0

[36] Sato G, Sekine K, Matsuda K, et al. Long-term prognosis of hearing loss in patients with unilateral Ménière's disease. Acta Oto-Laryngologica. 2014. DOI: 10.3109/00016489.2014.923114

[37] Seyed Tootoonchi SJ, Ghiasi S, Shadara P, Samani SM, Fouladi DF. Hearing function after betahistine therapy in patients with Ménière's disease. Brazilian Journal of Otorhinolaryngology. 2015. DOI: 10.1016/j.bjorl.2015.08.021

[38] Vernon J, Johnson R, Schleuning A. The characteristics and natural history of tinnitus in Meniere's disease. Otolaryngologic Clinics of North America. 1980. DOI: 10.1002/nur.20223

[39] Stouffer JL, Tyler RS. Characterization of tinnitus by tinnitus patients. The Journal of Speech and Hearing Disorders. 1990. DOI: 10.1044/jshd.5503.439

[40] Pfaltz C, Matefi L. Meniere's disease-or syndrome? A critical review of diagnose criteria. In: Vosteen K-H, Schuknecht H, Pfaltz C, et al., editors. Meniere's Disease, Pathogenesis, Diagnosis and Treatment. Stuttgart: Georg Thieme Verlag; 1981. pp. 1-10

[41] Paparella MM, Mancini F. Vestibular Meniere's disease. Otolaryngology-Head and Neck Surgery. 1985. DOI: 10.1177/019459988509300203

[42] Oosterveld W. Meniere's disease, signs and symptoms. The Journal of Laryngology and Otology. 1980;**94**(8): 885-892. DOI: 10.1017/S0022215100089647

[43] Silverstein H, Smouha E, Jones R. Natural history vs. surgery for Meniere's disease. Otolaryngology–Head and Neck Surgery. 1989. DOI: 10.1177/019459988910000102

[44] Tumarkin A. The otolithic catastrophe. British Medical Journal. 1936. DOI: 10.1136/bmj.2.3942.175

[45] Ödkvist LM, Bergenius J. Drop attacks in Meniere's disease. Acta Oto-Laryngologica, Suppl. 1988

[46] Oku R, Shigeno K, Kumagami H, Takahashi H. Otolith dysfunction during vertiginous attacks in Meniere's disease. Acta Oto-Laryngologica. 2003. DOI: 10.1080/00016480310000377

[47] Friberg U, Stahle J, Svedberg A. The natural course of Meniere's disease. Acta Oto-Laryngologica. 1983. DOI: 10.3109/00016488309123007

[48] Goebel JA. 2015 equilibrium committee amendment to the 1995 AAO-HNS guidelines for the definition of Ménière's disease. Otolaryngology–Head and Neck Surgery. 2016. DOI: 10.1177/0194599816628524

[49] Black FO, Kitch R. A review of vestibular test results in Meniere's disease. Otolaryngologic Clinics of North America. 1980. DOI: Pm: 18686702

[50] Maire R, Van Melle G. Vestibulo-ocular reflex characteristics in patients with unilateral Ménière's disease. Otology & Neurotology. 2008. DOI: 10.1097/MAO.0b013e3181776703

[51] Goin DW, Staller SJ, Asher DL, et al. Summating potential in Meniere's disease. The Laryngoscope. 1982. DOI: 10.3757/jser.55.419

[52] Klockhoff I. Diagnosis of Menière's disease. Archives of Oto-Rhino-Laryngology. 1976. DOI: 10.1007/BF00453679

[53] Rauch SD, Zhou G, Kujawa SG, Guinan JJ, Herrmann BS. Vestibular evoked myogenic potentials show altered tuning in patients with Ménière's disease. Otology & Neurotology. 2004. DOI: 10.1097/00129492-200405000-00022

[54] Nevoux J, Franco-Vidal V, Bouccara D, et al. Diagnostic and therapeutic strategy in Menière's disease. Guidelines of the French Otorhinolaryngology-Head and Neck Surgery Society (SFORL). European Annals of Otorhinolaryngology, Head and Neck Diseases. 2017;**134**(6):441-444. DOI: 10.1016/j.anorl.2016.12.003

[55] Van Esch BF, Van Der Zaag-Loonen HJ, Bruintjes TD, Van Benthem PPG. Interventions for Menière's disease: Protocol for an umbrella systematic review and a network meta-analysis. BMJ Open. 2016. DOI: 10.1136/bmjopen-2015-010269

[56] Hamill TA. Evaluating treatments for Meniere's disease: Controversies surrounding placebo control. Journal of the American Academy of Audiology. 2006. DOI: 10.3766/jaaa.17.1.4

[57] Torok N. Old and new in Ménière disease. The Laryngoscope. 1977. DOI: 10.1002/lary.1977.87.11.1870

[58] Green JD, Blum DJ, Harner SG. Longitudinal follow up of patients with Meniere's disease. Otolaryngology–Head and Neck Surgery. 1991. DOI: 10.1177/019459989110400603

[59] Nevoux J, Barbara M, Dornhoffer J, Gibson W, Kitahara T, Darrouzet V. International consensus (ICON) on treatment of Ménière's disease. European Annals of Otorhinolaryngology, Head and Neck Diseases. 2017. DOI: 10.1016/j.anorl.2017.12.006

[60] Holgers K-M, Finizia C. Health profiles for patients with Meniere's disease. Noise & Health. 2001

[61] Nakayama M, Masuda A, Ando KB, et al. A pilot study on the effi cacy of continuous positive airway pressure on the manifestations of Ménière's disease in patients with concomitant obstructive sleep apnea syndrome. Journal of Clinical Sleep Medicine. 2015. DOI: 10.5664/jcsm.5080

[62] Luxford E, Berliner KI, Lee J, Luxford WM. Dietary modification as adjunct treatment in Ménière's disease: Patient willingness and ability to comply. Otology & Neurotology. 2013. DOI: 10.1097/MAO.0b013e3182942261

[63] Sánchez-Sellero I, San-Román-Rodríguez E, Santos-Pérez S, Rossi-Izquierdo M, Soto-Varela A. Caffeine intake and Menière's disease: Is there relationship? Nutritional Neuroscience. 2017

[64] Coelho DH, Lalwani AK. Medical management of Ménière's disease. The Laryngoscope. 2008. DOI: 10.1097/MLG.0b013e31816927f0

[65] Sharon JD, Trevino C, Schubert MC, Carey JP. Treatment of Menière's disease. Current Treatment Options in Neurology. 2015;**17**(4). DOI: 10.1007/s11940-015- 0341-x

[66] He FJ, Li J, Macgregor GA. Effect of longer-term modest salt reduction on blood pressure. Cochrane Database of Systematic Reviews. 2013. DOI: 10.1002/14651858.CD004937.pub2

[67] Furuta H, Sato C, Kawaguchi Y, Miyashita T, Mori N. Expression of mRNAs encoding hormone receptors in

the endolymphatic sac of the rat. Acta Oto-Laryngologica. 1999. DOI: 10.1080/00016489950181936

[68] Kim G, Masilamani S, Turner R, et al. The thiazide-sensitive Na-Cl cotransporter is an aldosterone-induced protein. Proceedings of the National Academy of Sciences of the United States of America. 1998. DOI: 10.1093/icb/23.2.347

[69] Rossier BC, Baker ME, Studer RA. Epithelial sodium transport and its control by aldosterone: The story of our internal environment revisited. Physiological Reviews. 2015. DOI: 10.1152/physrev.00011.2014

[70] Miyashita T, Tatsumi H, Hayakawa K, Mori N, Sokabe M. Large Na+ influx and high Na+, K+-ATPase activity in mitochondria-rich epithelial cells of the inner ear endolymphatic sac. Pflügers Archiv - European Journal of Physiology. 2007. DOI: 10.1007/s00424-006-0166-2

[71] Akiyama K, Miyashita T, Mori T, Inamoto R, Mori N. Expression of thiazide-sensitive Na+-Cl- cotransporter in the rat endolymphatic sac. Biochemical and Biophysical Research Communications. 2008. DOI: 10.1016/j.bbrc.2008.04.081

[72] Kim SH, Park HY, Choi HS, Chung HP, Choi JY. Functional and molecular expression of epithelial sodium channels in cultured human endolymphatic sac epithelial cells. Otology & Neurotology. 2009. DOI: 10.1097/MAO.0b013e31819a8e0e

[73] Matsubara A, Miyashita T, Inamoto R, Hoshikawa H, Mori N. Cystic fibrosis transmembrane conductance regulator in the endolymphatic sac of the rat. Auris, Nasus, Larynx. 2014. DOI: 10.1016/j.anl.2014.02.005

[74] Mori N, Uozumi N, Yura K, Sakai SI. Effect of aldosterone antagonist on the DC potential in the endolymphatic SAC. The Annals of Otology, Rhinology, and Laryngology. 1991. DOI: 10.1177/000348949110000112

[75] Mori N, Uozumi N, Yura K, Sakai S. The difference in endocochlear and endolymphatic sac d.c. potentials in response to furosemide and canrenoate as diuretics. European Archives of Oto-Rhino-Laryngology. 1990. DOI: 10.1007/BF00179010

[76] Thai-Van H, Bounaix MJ, Fraysse B. Menière's disease: Pathophysiology and treatment. Drugs. 2001. DOI: 10.2165/00003495-200161080-00005

[77] Miyashita T, Inamoto R, Fukuda S, et al. Hormonal changes following a low-salt diet in patients with Ménière's disease. Auris, Nasus, Larynx. 2017; **44**(1):52-57. DOI: 10.1016/j.anl.2016.03.001

[78] Tadros SF, Frisina ST, Mapes F, Frisina DR, Frisina RD. Higher serum aldosterone correlates with lower hearing thresholds: A possible protective hormone against presbycusis. Hearing Research. 2005. DOI: 10.1016/j.heares.2005.05.009

[79] Martinez DM. The effect of serc (betahistine hydrochloride) on the circulation of the inner ear in experimental animals. Acta Oto-Laryngologica. 1972. DOI: 10.3109/00016487209122697

[80] Lacour M, van de Heyning PH, Novotny M, Tighilet B. Betahistine in the treatment of Ménière's disease. Neuropsychiatric Disease and Treatment. 2007

[81] Timmerman H. Pharmacotherapy of vertigo: Any news to be expected? Acta Oto-Laryngologica. 1994. DOI: 10.3109/00016489409127323

[82] Betahistine dihydrochloride. Electronic Medicines Compendium.

2015. Available from: https://www.medicines.org.uk/emc/medicine/266172015

[83] Murdin L, Hussain K, Schilder AGM. Betahistine for symptoms of vertigo. Cochrane Database of Systematic Reviews. 2013. DOI: 10.1002/14651858.CD010696

[84] Nauta JJP. Meta-analysis of clinical studies with betahistine in Ménière's disease and vestibular vertigo. European Archives of Oto-Rhino-Laryngology. 2014. DOI: 10.1007/s00405-013-2596-8

[85] Adrion C, Fischer CS, Wagner J, Gürkov R, Mansmann U, Strupp M. Efficacy and safety of betahistine treatment in patients with Meniere's disease: Primary results of a long term, multicentre, double blind, randomised, placebo controlled, dose defining trial (BEMED trial). BMJ. 2016;**352**. DOI: 10.1136/bmj.h6816

[86] Shinkawa H, Kimura RS. Effect of diuretics on endolymphatic hydrops. Acta Oto-Laryngologica. 1986. DOI: 10.3109/00016488609108606

[87] Petermann W, Mulch G. Long-term therapy of Meniere's disease. Comparison of the effects of betahistine dihydrochloride and hydrochlorothiazide. Fortschritte der Medizin. 1982

[88] Van Deelen GW, Huizing EH. Use of a diuretic (Dyazide®) in the treatment of ménière's disease: A double-blind cross-over placebo-controlled study. ORL; Journal for Oto-rhino-laryngology and its Related Specialties. 1986. DOI: 10.1159/000275884

[89] Klockhoff I, Lindblom U. Meniére's disease and hydrochlorothiazide dichlotride®—A critical analysis of symptoms and therapeutic effects. Acta Oto-Laryngologica. 1967. DOI: 10.3109/00016486709128769

[90] Thirlwall AS, Kundu S. Diuretics for Meniere's disease or syndrome. Cochrane Database of Systematic Reviews. 2006. DOI: 10.1002/14651858.CD003599.pub2

[91] Ingelstedt S, Ivarsson A, Tjernström Ö. Immediate relief of symptoms during acute attacks of Meniere's disease, using a pressure chamber. Acta Oto-Laryngologica. 1976. DOI: 10.3109/00016487609120921

[92] Gates GA, Green JD, Tucci DL, Telian SA. The effects of transtympanic micropressure treatment in people with unilateral Ménière's disease. Archives of Otolaryngology – Head & Neck Surgery. 2004. DOI: 10.1001/archotol.130.6.718

[93] Ahsan SF, Standring R, Wang Y. Systematic review and meta–Analysis of Meniett therapy for Meniere's disease. The Laryngoscope. 2015;**125**(1):203-208. DOI: 10.1002/lary.24773

[94] Syed MI, Rutka JA, Hendry J, Browning GG. Positive pressure therapy for Meniere's syndrome/disease with a Meniett device: A systematic review of randomised controlled trials. Clinical Otolaryngology. 2015. DOI: 10.1111/coa.12344

[95] van Sonsbeek S, Pullens B, van Benthem PP. Positive pressure therapy for Ménière's disease or syndrome. Cochrane Database of Systematic Reviews. 2015. DOI: 10.1002/14651858.CD008419.pub2

[96] Zhang S-L, Leng Y, Liu B, Shi H, Lu M, Kong W-J. Meniett therapy for Meniere's disease: An updated Meta-analysis. Otology & Neurotology. 2016;**37**(3):290-298. DOI: 10.1097/MAO.0000000000000957

[97] Sugawara K, Kitamura K, Ishida T, Sejima T. Insertion of tympanic ventilation tubes as a treating modality for patients with Meniere's disease: A short- and long-term follow-up study in

seven cases. Auris, Nasus, Larynx. 2003. DOI: 10.1016/S0385-8146(02)00105-0

[98] Montandon PB, Guillemin P, Häusler R. Prevention of vertigo in Mèniér's syndrome by means of transtympanic ventilation tubes. ORL: Journal for Oto-rhino-laryngology and its Related Specialties. 1988. DOI: 10.1159/000276016

[99] Ballester M, Liard P, Vibert D, Häusler R. Menière's disease in the elderly. Otology & Neurotology. 2002

[100] Ogawa Y, Otsuka K, Hagiwara A, et al. Clinical study of tympanostomy tube placement for patients with intractable Ménière's disease. The Journal of Laryngology and Otology. 2015;**129**(2):120-125. DOI: 10.1017/S0022215115000079

[101] Masutani H, Nakai Y, Kato A. Microvascular disorder of the stria vascularis in endolymphatic hydrops. Acta Oto-Laryngologica. 1995. DOI: 10.3109/00016489509121874

[102] Yazawa Y, Kitano H, Suzuki M, Tanaka H, Kitajima K. Studies of cochlear blood flow in Guinea pigs with endolymphatic hydrops. ORL; Journal for Oto-rhino-laryngology and its Related Specialties. 1998. DOI: 10.1159/000027554

[103] Kimura RS, Hutta J. Inhibition of experimentally induced endolymphatic hydrops by middle ear ventilation. European Archives of Oto-Rhino-Laryngology. 1997. DOI: 10.1007/BF00874091

[104] Chi FL, Liang Q, Wang ZM. Effects of hyperbaric therapy on function and morphology of Guinea pig cochlea with endolymphatic hydrops. Otology & Neurotology. 2004. DOI: 10.1097/00129492-200407000-00024

[105] Dornhoffer JL, King D. The effect of the Meniett device in patients with Ménière's disease: Long-term results. Otology & Neurotology. 2008. DOI: 10.1097/MAO.0b013e318182025a

[106] Foster CA. Optimal management of Ménière's disease. Therapeutics and Clinical Risk Management. 2015. DOI: 10.2147/TCRM.S59023

[107] Peterson WM, Isaacson JE. Current management of Ménière's disease in an only hearing ear. Otology & Neurotology. 2007;**28**(5):696-699. DOI: 10.1097/mao.0b013e3180577963

[108] Tumarkin A. Thoughts on the treatment of labyrinthopathy. The Journal of Laryngology and Otology;**80**(10):1041-1053. DOI: 10.1017/S0022215100066366

[109] Lall M. Meniere's disease and the grommet (survey of its therapeutic effects). The Journal of Laryngology and Otology. 1977;**83**(8):787-791. DOI: 10.1017/S002221510007095X

[110] Cinnamond MJ. Eustachian tube function in Meniére's disease. The Journal of Laryngology and Otology. 1975. DOI: 10.1017/S0022215100080075

[111] Hall CM, Brackmann DE. Eustachian tube blockage and Meniere's disease. Archives of Otolaryngology – Head & Neck Surgery. 1977;**103**(6):355-357. DOI: 10.1001/archotol.1977.00780230077012

[112] Thomsen J, Bonding P, Birgit B. The non-specific effect of endolymphatic sac surgery in treatment of Meniere's disease: A prospective, randomized controlled study comparing "classic" endolymphatic sac surgery with the insertion of a ventilating tube in the tympanic membrane. Acta Oto-Laryngologica. 1998;**118**(6):769-773. DOI: 10.1080/00016489850182413

[113] Magnan J, Ozgirgin ON, Trabalzini F, et al. European position statement on diagnosis, and treatment of Meniere's

disease*. The Journal of International Advanced Otology. 2018;**14**(2):317-321. DOI: 10.5152/iao.2018.140818

[114] Guneri EA. Endolenfatik hidrops ve Meniere hastaligi. In: Onerci M, editor. Kulak Burun Boğaz Baş Boyun Cerrahisi Cilt 2 Nörootoloji. Ankara: Matsa Basimevi; 2016. pp. 523-536

[115] Bienhold H, Flohr H. Role of cholinergic synapses in vestibular compensation. Brain Research. 1980. DOI: 10.1016/0006-8993(80)90083-9

[116] Ishikawa K, Igarashi M. Effect of diazepam on vestibular compensation in squirrel monkeys. Archives of Oto-Rhino-Laryngology. 1984. DOI: 10.1007/BF00464344

[117] Schaefer K, Meyer D. Aspects of vestibular compensation in Guinea pig. In: Flohr H, Precht E, editors. Lesion-Induced Neuronal Plasticity in Sensorimotor System. New York: Springer; 1981. pp. 197-297

[118] Antor MA, Uribe AA, Erminy-Falcon N, et al. The effect of transdermal scopolamine for the prevention of postoperative nausea and vomiting. Frontiers in Pharmacology. 2014. DOI: 10.3389/fphar.2014.00055

[119] Gejrot T. Intravenous xylocaine in the treatment of attacks of Meniere's disease. Acta Oto-Laryngologica. 1976. DOI: 10.3109/00016487609120911

[120] Orji F. The influence of psychological factors in Meniere's disease. Annals of Medical and Health Sciences Research. 2014;**4**(1):3. DOI: 10.4103/2141-9248.126601

[121] Van Cruijsen N, Wit H, Albers F. Psychological aspects of Ménière's disease. Acta Oto-Laryngologica. 2003. DOI: 10.1080/0036554021000028125

[122] House JW, Crary WG, Wexler M. The inter-relationship of vertigo and stress. Otolaryngologic Clinics of North America. 1980

[123] Eagger S, Luxon LM, Davies RA, Coelho A, Ron MA. Psychiatric morbidity in patients with peripheral vestibular disorder: A clinical and neuro-otological study. Journal of Neurology, Neurosurgery, and Psychiatry. 1992. DOI: 10.1136/jnnp.55.5.383

[124] Takahashi M, Ishida K, Iida M, Yamashita H, Sugawara K. Analysis of lifestyle and behavioral characteristics in Ménière's disease patients and a control population. Acta Oto-Laryngologica. 2001. DOI: 10.1080/000164801300043721

[125] Van Cruijsen N, Jaspers JPC, Van De Wiel HBM, Wit HP, Albers FWJ. Psychological assessment of patients with Menière's disease. International Journal of Audiology. 2006. DOI: 10.1080/14992020600753239

[126] Yokota Y, Kitahara T, Sakagami M, et al. Surgical results and psychological status in patients with intractable Ménière's disease. Auris, Nasus, Larynx. 2016;**43**(3):287-291. DOI: 10.1016/j.anl.2015.10.007

[127] Dowdal-Osborn M. Early vestibular rehabilitation in patients with Meniere's disease. Otolaryngologic Clinics of North America. 2002;**35**(3):683-690. DOI: 10.1016/S0030-6665(02)00026-9

[128] Di Fabio RP. Sensitivity and specificity of platform posturography for identifying patients with vestibular dysfunction. Physical Therapy. 1995. DOI: 10.1093/ptj/75.4.290

[129] Black FO, Wall C. Comparison of vestibulo-ocular and vestibulospinal screening tests. Otolaryngology-Head and Neck Surgery. 1981. DOI: 10.1177/019459988108900523

[130] Di Fabio RP. Meta-analysis of the sensitivity and specificity of platform

posturography. Archives of Otolaryngology – Head & Neck Surgery. 1996. DOI: 10.1001/archotol.1996.01890140036008

[131] Cohen H, Ewell LR, Jenkins HA. Disability in Meniere's disease. Archives of Otolaryngology-Head and Neck Surgery. 1995. DOI: 10.1001/archotol.1995.01890010017004

[132] Haybach P. Meniere's disease—What you need to know. In: Vestibular Disorders Association. Portland, Oregon; 1998

[133] Odkvist L. Gentamicin cures Vertigo, but what happens to hearing? The International Tinnitus Journal. 1997

[134] Gottshall K, Hoffer ME, Kopke R. Vestibular physical therapy rehabilitation after low dose microcatheter administered gentamicin treatment for Meniere's disease. In: 4th International Symposium on Meniere's Disease. Hauge (Netherlands): Kuglar Publications; 2000. pp. 663-668

[135] Suryanarayanan R, Cook JA. Long-term results of gentamicin inner ear perfusion in Ménière's disease. The Journal of Laryngology and Otology. 2004. DOI: 10.1258/0022215041615083

[136] Clendaniel RA, Tucci DL. Vestibular rehabilitation strategies in Meniere's disease. Otolaryngologic Clinics of North America. 1997

[137] Gottshall KR, Topp SG, Hoffer ME. Early vestibular physical therapy rehabilitation for Meniere's disease. Otolaryngologic Clinics of North America. 2010;**43**(5):1113-1119. DOI: 10.1016/j.otc.2010.05.006

[138] Cohen H. Vestibular rehabilitation improves daily life function. American Journal of Occupational Therapy. 1994. DOI: 10.1097/IGC.0b013e31828b4f19

[139] Antoli Candela F Jr. The histopathology of Meniere's disease. Acta Oto-Laryngologica. 1976

[140] Lee CS, Paparella MM, Margolis RH, Le C. Audiological profiles and Meniere's disease. Ear, Nose, & Throat Journal. 1995

[141] Stahle J, Friberg U, Svedberg A. Long-term progression of Meniere's disease. Acta Oto-Laryngologica. 1991. DOI: 10.3109/00016489109128047

[142] Kolbe U, Brehmer D, Schaaf H, Hesse G, Laubert A. Tinnitus and morbus Meniere. In: Sterkers O, Ferrary E, Dauman R, Sauvage JP, Tran Ba Huy P, editors. Meniere's Disease 1999-Update. Kugler Publications; 2000. pp. 459-462

[143] Vasama JP, Linthicum FH. Meniere's disease and endolymphatic hydrops without Meniere's symptoms: Temporal bone histopathology. Acta Oto-Laryngologica. 1999. DOI: 10.1080/00016489950181279

[144] Sala T. Transtympanic gentamicin in the treatment of Meniére's disease. Auris, Nasus, Larynx. 1997

[145] Kaasinen S, Pyykkö I, Ishizaki H, Aalto H. Effect of intratympanically administered gentamicin on hearing and tinnitus in Meniere's disease. Acta Oto-Laryngologica. 1995. DOI: 10.3109/00016489509125223

[146] Ganança MM, Caovilla HH, Gazzola JM, Ganança CF, Ganança FF. Betahistine in the treatment of tinnitus in patients with vestibular disorders. Brazilian Journal of Otorhinolaryngology. 2011. DOI: 10.1590/S1808-86942011000400014

[147] Azevedo AA, Figueiredo RR, Elgoyhen AB, Langguth B, Penido NDO, Schlee W. Tinnitus treatment with oxytocin: A pilot study. Frontiers in

Neurology. 2017. DOI: 10.3389/fneur.2017.00494

[148] Langguth B, Kreuzer PM, Kleinjung T, De Ridder D. Tinnitus: Causes and clinical management. Lancet Neurology. 2013. DOI: 10.1016/S1474-4422(13)70160-1

[149] Perez R, Chen JM, Nedzelski JM. The status of the contralateral ear in established unilateral Menière's disease. The Laryngoscope. 2004. DOI: 10.1097/00005537-200408000-00010

[150] Yazawa Y, Kitahara M. Bilateral endolymphatic hydrops in Meniere's disease: Review of temporal bone autopsies. The Annals of Otology, Rhinology, and Laryngology. 1990. DOI: 10.1177/000348949009900705

[151] Tsuji K, Velazquez-Villasenor L, Rauch S, Glynn R, Wall CI, Merchant S. Temporal bone studies of the human peripheral vestibular system. Meniere's disease. The Annals of Otology, Rhinology, and Laryngology. 2000. DOI: 10.1177/00034894001090S502

[152] Kitahara M. Bilateral aspects of Meniere's disease: Meniere's disease with bilateral fluctuant hearing loss. Acta Oto-Laryngologica. 1991. DOI: 10.3109/00016489109128046

[153] Agrawal S, Parnes L. Systemic treatment of bilateral Meniere's disease. In: Roland P, Rutka J, editors. Ototoxicity. Hamilton, Canada: BC Decker; 2004

[154] Mizuta K, Furuta M, Ito Y, et al. A case of Meniere's disease with vertical nystagmus after administration of glycerol. Auris, Nasus, Larynx. 2000. DOI: 10.1016/S0385-8146(00)00050-X

[155] Paparella MM, Griebie MS. Bilaterality of Meniere's disease. Acta Oto-Laryngologica. 1984. DOI: 10.3109/00016488409130984

[156] Iseli C, Gibson W. A comparison of three methods of using transtympanic electrocochleography for the diagnosis of Meniere's disease: Click summating potential measurements, tone burst summating potential amplitude measurements, and biasing of the summating potential using a low frequency tone. Acta Oto-Laryngologica. 2010. DOI: 10.3109/00016480902858899

[157] Lin MY, Timmer FCA, Oriel BS, et al. Vestibular evoked myogenic potentials (VEMP) can detect asymptomatic saccular hydrops. The Laryngoscope. 2006. DOI: 10.1097/01.mlg.0000216815.75512.03

[158] Fukuoka H, Tsukada K, Miyagawa M, et al. Semi-quantitative evaluation of endolymphatic hydrops by bilateral intratympanic gadolinium-based contrast agent (GBCA) administration with MRI for Meniere's disease. Acta Oto-Laryngologica. 2010. DOI: 10.3109/00016480902858881

[159] Garduño-Anaya MA, De Toledo HC, Hinojosa-González R, Pane-Pianese C, Ríos-Castañeda LC. Dexamethasone inner ear perfusion by intratympanic injection in unilateral Ménière's disease: A two-year prospective, placebo-controlled, double-blind, randomized trial. Otolaryngology-Head and Neck Surgery. 2005. DOI: 10.1016/j.otohns.2005.05.010

[160] Silverstein H, Isaacson JE, Olds MJ, Rowan PT, Rosenberg S. Dexamethasone inner ear perfusion for the treatment of Meniere's disease: A prospective, randomized, double-blind, crossover trial. American Journal of Otolaryngology. 1998. DOI: 10.1111/j.1467-6494.1954.tb02338.x

[161] Alles MJRC, Der Gaag MA, Stokroos RJ. Intratympanic steroid therapy for inner ear diseases, a review of the literature. European Archives of

Oto-Rhino-Laryngology. 2006. DOI: 10.1007/s00405-006-0065-3

[162] Balyan FR, Taibah A, De Donato G, et al. Titration streptomycin therapy in Meniere's disease: Long-term results. Otolaryngology-Head and Neck Surgery. 1998. DOI: 10.1016/S0194-5998(98)80028-4

[163] Graham MD. Bilateral Meniere's disease. Treatment with intramuscular titration streptomycin sulfate. Otolaryngologic Clinics of North America. 1997

[164] Kilpatrick JK, Sismanis A, Spencer RF, Wise CM. Low-dose oral methotrexate management of patients with bilateral Meniere's disease. Ear, Nose, & Throat Journal. 2000

[165] Schessel D, Minor L, Nedzelski J. Meniere's disease and other peripheral vestibular disorders. In: Cummings C, Flint P, Haughey B, editors. Cummings Otolaryngology: Head and Neck Surgery. 4th ed. Philadelphia: Elsevier Inc; 2005

[166] Shea JJJ, Ge X. Dexamethasone perfusion of the labyrinth plus intravenous dexamethasone for Meniere's disease. Otolaryngologic Clinics of North America. 1996

[167] Shea JJ. The role of dexamethasone or streptomycin perfusion in the treatment of Meniere's disease. Otolaryngologic Clinics of North America. 1997

[168] Hirvonen TP, Peltomaa M, Ylikoski J. Intratympanic and systemic dexamethasone for Meniere's disease. ORL; Journal for Oto-rhino-laryngology and its Related Specialties. 2000. DOI: 10.1159/000027730

[169] Morales-Luckie E, Cornejo-Suarez A, Zaragoza-Contreras MA, Gonzalez-Perez O. Oral administration of prednisone to control refractory vertigo in Ménière's disease: A pilot study. Otology & Neurotology. 2005. DOI: 10.1097/01.mao.0000185057.81962.51

[170] Paparella M. Revision of endolymphatic sac surgery for recurrent Meniere's disease. Otolaryngologic Clinics of North America. 2002;**35**(3): 607-619. DOI: 10.1016/S0030-6665(02)00032-4

[171] Kitahara T, Kubo T, Okumura SI, Kitahara M. Effects of endolymphatic sac drainage with steroids for intractable Ménière's disease: A long-term follow-up and randomized controlled study. The Laryngoscope. 2008. DOI: 10.1097/MLG.0b013e3181651c4a

[172] Wetmore SJ. Endolymphatic sac surgery for Ménière's disease: Long-term results after primary and revision surgery. Archives of Otolaryngology – Head & Neck Surgery. 2008. DOI: 10.1001/archotol.134.11.1144

Section 4

Intratympanic Treatment for Meniere's Disease

Chapter 4

The Treatment of Meniere's Disease by the Intratympanic Therapy

Maria Stella A. Amaral, Henrique F. Pauna, Ana Claudia M.B. Reis and Miguel A. Hyppolito

Abstract

Meniere's disease represents one of the most frequent vestibulopathy, with prevalence of 46–200 cases per 100,000, without difference between genders and manifests in fourth decade of life. Features include dizziness/vertigo, hearing loss, tinnitus, and ear fullness. Individuals with Meniere's disease have poor quality of life due to dizziness, regarding physical, functional, and emotional aspects. The therapeutic measures are proposed, depending on the stage of the disease. About 95% of the patients are well controlled with conservative clinical treatment. The remaining 5% have incapacitating symptoms. These patients are candidates for surgical treatments classics, decompression of the endolymphatic sac, vestibular neurectomy, or labyrinthectomy. Intratympanic gentamicin injections emerged as an alternative to surgical treatments, whose risk and benefit ratio has been shown to be much more satisfactory. Aminoglycosides, such as gentamicin have been used since the decade of 1950 for the vestibular chemical ablation in cases of intractable vertigo. The drawback is that gentamicin causes irreversible destruction to cochlear hair cells with hearing loss. The selective vestibulotoxicity in the treatment of Meniere's disease can be used in the treatment of the vertigo promoting a chemical labyrinthectomy.

Keywords: Meniere's disease, vestibulopathy, vertigo treatment, chemical labyrinthectomy, vestibulotoxicity

1. Introduction

Meniere's disease (MD) is a clinical entity characterized by episodic vertigo, fluctuant sensorineural hearing loss (SNHL), tinnitus, and a pressure sensation of the ear. It can happen uni- or bilaterally, and diagnosis is made clinically, according to the classification of the American Academy of Otolaryngology—Head and Neck Surgery, updated in 2015 (**Table 1**) [1, 2]. MD is a chronic condition affecting about 190/100,000 patients in US, a general incidence about 50–200/100,000 per year, and a lower incidence of 17/100,000 per year in Japan [3].

The diagnosis of MD remains eminently clinical and its manifestations are widely variable. Many patients have audiological symptoms, some have mainly vestibular complaints and few patients have a combination of auditory and vestibular symptoms. The bilateral involvement can be observed in 10–50% of the patients, which leads to a condition difficult to treat and with unfavorable prognosis [4].

Definite	Two or more episodes of vertigo* plus audiometrically confirmed low- to medium-frequency SNHL in one ear on at least one occasion before, during, or after one of the episodes of vertigo; fluctuating aural symptoms** in the affected ear; not better accounted for by another vestibular diagnosis
Probable	Two or more episodes of vertigo or dizziness, each lasting 20 min to 24 h; fluctuating aural symptoms** in the affected ear; other causes excluded

*Defined as spontaneous, rotational vertigo lasting 20 min to 12 h.
**Hearing, tinnitus, or fullness.*

Table 1.
Criteria of diagnosis of MD.

2. Otopathology

Prosper Meniere, who worked as a director of the first school for the deaf-mute in Paris, described in 1861, a combination of vertigo, imbalance, and hearing impairment reflecting an inner ear disease [1]. But, only in 1937, with the discovery of endolymphatic hydrops (EH) in human temporal bones by Yamakawa and Hallpike and Cairns, the pathologic displacement of Reissner's membrane into the scala vestibuli—and so with the dilation of the scala media of the cochlea—was first stablished (**Figure 1**) [5].

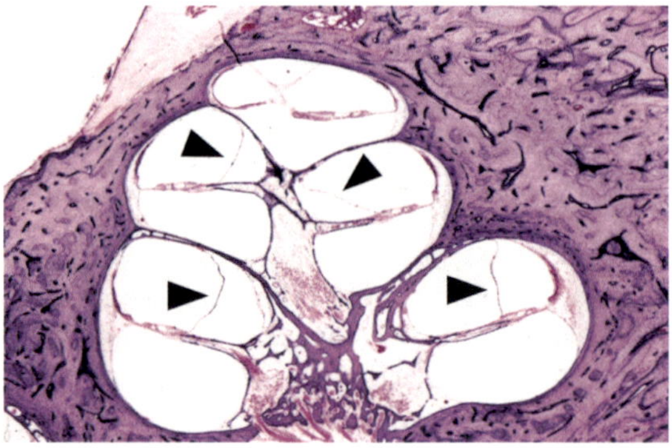

Figure 1.
Reissner's membrane displaced in a temporal bone with hydrops (arrowheads).

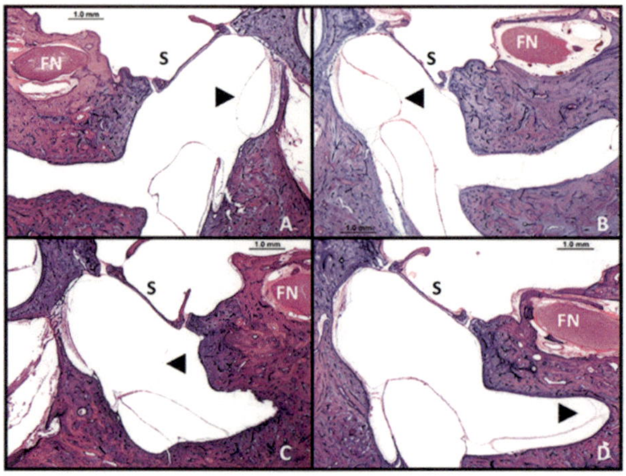

Figure 2.
Membranous structures displaced in MD. The arrowhead points the membranous structure called saccule, in different stages of hydrops (A, normal; B, slight; C, moderate; and D, severe). FN-facial nerve; S-stapes.

Many other disorders can be related with hydrops, as aforementioned: temporal bone fracture, otosclerosis, diabetes mellitus, syphilis, hormonal disorders, migraine, and others. Diseases that can cause MD are as follows: food allergy, dyslipidemia, and autoimmune diseases [3, 6]. These disorders can also affect inner ear composition and displace in various degrees other membranous structures, including saccule, utricle, and the ampullae of the semicircular canals (**Figure 2**) [5].

3. Audiological findings

Several tests and evaluation methods have been employed for the diagnosis of MD. These include audiological tests, vestibular, radiological, clinical, and biochemical parameters. However, the lack of a definitive diagnostic test makes the process of diagnosis sometimes longer or frustrating. For this reason, the professional should be well experienced in the decision of when and what test should be used for the diagnostic process and, especially, to know how to interpret the results [7].

Although MD is not a rare condition, there is a delay in the diagnosis. Probably this is due to factors such as the difficulty of the differential diagnosis between other inner ear diseases, mainly due to the occurrence of nonspecific symptoms in the early stages of the disease and the absence of specific tests, in addition to the floating characteristic of MD which hinders the interpretation of the tests [8].

Patients with hearing loss and balance disorders are commonly diagnosed as having MD, which sometimes characterizes a diagnostic error, due to the lack of specific diagnostic tests [7, 8].

The main objective of early diagnosis is the early intervention, aiming to reduce the frequency and intensity of the crisis of vertigo and, at the same time, to preserve the hearing and vestibular functions [7]. Nonetheless, it is common among patients with MD, psychological suffering and loss in quality of life due to the crisis of vertigo [9, 10].

Some procedures significantly collaborate for the diagnosis of MD; however, it is important to emphasize the correlation of clinical history and symptoms with the results of the behavioral evaluation and testing goals for the conclusion of the case. In MD, a progressive hearing loss occurs with disappearance of vertigo in 70% of cases.

In addition, the audiological evaluation is important in monitoring treatment, as in the case of chemistry labyrinthectomy with gentamicin.

Tonal threshold audiometry is the basic examination used in the process of diagnosis and follow-up of MD and has a decisive role in treatment decisions. The progressive sensorineural hearing loss, with impairment of low frequencies and the fluctuations, is typical result observed in MD.

The degree of hearing loss seems to be related to the stage of the disease and has a relationship with the symptomatic period. It is common for MD patients a sensorineural hearing loss to moderate to severe before or on the first diagnosis. The settings of the hearing loss may vary; the most common is the ascendant or inverted "U." The flat configuration appears in more advanced stages of the disease. However, different audiometric results can be found and variations in the degree and configuration of hearing loss may be observed, depending on the stage of the disease. Although the low frequencies are generally more affected, hearing loss may be present in all frequencies when in an advanced state of the disease, configuring sometimes an audiogram with flat curve [11]. In this way, the diagnosis of MD should not be established in accordance with the configuration of the audiogram, because there is not a specific audiometric pattern [12]. There is no consensus in the literature that the auditory thresholds for pure tone should be investigated, including thresholds of air and bone conduction and, at least for the frequencies 250 Hz–8 kHz. A difference ≥10 dB is accepted as the float hearing for the MD.

Relationship was found between the occurrence of fluctuation and the severity or progression of the hearing loss. Authors report that the hearing losses affecting the averages (between 500 and 2000 Hz) and high frequencies (between 3000 and 8000 Hz) suggest a worse prognosis than that one affects the low frequencies (between 125 and 500 Hz) [13]. The value of the results of the hearing evaluation by means of ATL has been shown to be significant, and the cochlear symptoms have been described in the literature as the most common initial sign of the disease and, many times, to appear before the vertigo.

The speech perception tests are also compromised. The percentage index of speech recognition (PISR) and the speech recognition threshold (SRT) are altered in MD [12, 13]. The average score of the PISR, when there is hearing loss can be around 56% or less if the MD is of long duration. In cases of unilateral hearing loss, percentages of PISR worst in relation to expected, considering the results of the auditory thresholds for pure tone. The speech in noise tests has helped in the intervention of the patients with MD; individuals with MD unilaterally submitted to simultaneous labyrinthectomy have improvement in sound localization and in speech understanding with and without competitive noise [13]. Acoustic immittance measures course with a type A configuration tympanometry, although in some patients with severe hearing loss of long term may present tympanometry curve characteristic of tubal dysfunction. The acoustic reflex threshold decreases in cochlear pathologies due to recruitment, the difference between the acoustic reflex thresholds of the frequencies of 500, 1000, and 2000 Hz and the tonal auditory thresholds obtained by air, the same frequencies of 60 dB or less, and outcome goal that suggests the presence of cochlear pathology (recruitment) [13]. It is worth mentioning that the acoustic immittance measures can be very useful in the diagnosis of MD, in cases of MD floating and nonfloating and with respect to the prediction of endolymphatic hydrops reversible and irreversible.

Electrocochleography (ECochG) can be used for MD diagnosis. The presence of endolymphatic hydrops is determined by the enlargement of the summation potential (SP) in relation to the action potential (AP), reflecting an increase in relation SP/AP. The SP enlargement is more evident when the patient presents fullness and mild hearing loss. In the initial stages of the MD, the increase in the endolymphatic volume alters the hydromechanical properties of cochlear stretching medium scale and changing SP. The specificity of the relationship SP/AP is larger than the sensitivity in MD. The increase of SP/AP relationship suggests the diagnosis of MD, but only in about 50% of the cases, the disease really exists [13].

4. Available treatments

The characteristics of the MD are well documented, as well as the treatments for this pathology. The available literature is focused to identify the etiology and how to clinically approach the symptomatic patient. The symptomatic treatment can be pharmacological and/or surgical.

The symptomatic treatment does not prevent the progression of the disease. This treatment may involve diet, vestibular therapy, and drug treatment [11]. In acute vertigo crisis, drugs that block the vestibular reflexes in the vestibule-cerebral shaft can be used. They are chlorpromazine, cinnarizine, promethazine, and diazepam [5, 14].

The endolymphatic hydrops found in MD is treated aiming to prevent its progression. In this way, there is a low sodium diet and use of diuretics, such as furosemide and hydrochlorothiazide [6].

Vasodilators are used for long-term treatment based on the fact that the hydrops can be caused by ischemia of the stria vascularis. Currently, the medical treatment of maintenance is betahistine with or without diuretic [6, 10].

5. Symptomatic chemical-surgical treatment

Studies have shown that the toxic effects of aminoglycosides in the sensorineural epithelium of the inner ear, particularly in the labyrinth, can be considered as a therapy for MD [6, 10].

In cases of MD with bilateral vestibular symptoms is difficult to control and with important hearing loss, has already been given in the past to ablation of the maze with systemic aminoglycosides because they control the vertigo. However, the cumulative doses of aminoglycosides increase the risk of ototoxicity with permanent cochlear damage and the possibility of causing ataxia and oscillopsia. Currently, with the possibility of injecting substances via transtympanic route, the indications for systemic use of aminoglycosides are limited [15].

6. Surgical treatment

In about 70% of the cases, MD evolves to progressive hearing loss with improvement to the vestibular symptoms. For the other 30% who do not present an improvement of vestibular symptoms, even with the clinical treatment, surgical treatment should be thought.

The decision to operate and the choice of procedure are often dictated by the understanding and experience of each surgeon [3]. Surgical treatment to be considered varies from conservative to destructive, depending on whether or not there is a hearing loss [3]. The surgery that is the most popular is the endolymphatic sac decompression, and it is known as a conservative surgical procedure and is widely accepted.

This surgery was first described by Portmann, in 1927, but the precise role by which the surgery works remains undefined [16]. Among the destructive surgical treatments, we have a vestibular neurectomy, the cochleo-sacculotomy, the transcanal labyrinthectomy, or postauricular labyrinthectomy [4].

7. Transtympanic treatment

The use of systemic aminoglycosides was replaced by intratympanic gentamycin instillations that are administered once a day by a limited number of days. The intratympanic administration of drugs for the treatment of the MD was primarily described by Schuknecht in 1957 [17]. The intratympanic injections of gentamicin provide a high rate of success in the control of vertigo with reduced number of side effects on hearing [18, 19].

The intratympanic injections of gentamicin were proposed by Stokroos. After anesthesia of the tympanic membrane, gentamicin is administered in the middle ear through a fine needle of lumbar puncture in a fixed dose of 30 mg/ml [20, 21].

One other substance that can be used is steroid, which may decrease the inflammatory reaction in the inner ear, thus decreasing the endolymphatic hydrops. It has been reported that the use of corticosteroids may help to control the inner ear dysfunction, thereby decreasing vestibular symptoms up to 91% of MD patients (with 1–4 injections of dexamethasone at a concentration of 12 mg/ml) [22, 23].

Another substance to be injected is methylprednisolone, with higher concentrations and with the possibility to last longer in the perilymph. However, many authors described data suggesting same effectiveness of both steroids [24, 25].

Both gentamicin and steroids are absorbed by perilymph through the round window membrane (which is semipermeable), the annular ligament of the oval window, and by the small lacunar mesh that surrounds the inner ear [25].

A randomized, double-blind controlled study compared the use of transtympanic gentamicin (40 mg/ml) and corticosteroids (methylprednisolone [62.5 mg/ml]), and no difference was observed regarding the effectiveness of both groups of treatments [26].

8. Injection protocols

1. Patient positioned at supine position;

2. Head is positioned in a slightly hyper-extension with 30° contralateral rotation;

3. Instillation 2% lidocaine in ear canal, removing completely after 15 min;

4. Under microscopic examination, tympanic membrane is anesthetized with 80–90% phenol solution at inferior and posterior tympanic membrane quadrant;

5. In few minutes, the transtympanic access could be performed using a spinal needle and a flexible catheter mounted on an insulin syringe;

6. Slow instillations of 1 ml of 26–40 mg/ml, not buffered with bicarbonate sodium in two 0.5 ml injection with 30 min apart;

7. Patient remained motionless for 30 min.

This protocol can be repeated each week or monthly for six times.

To maintain auditory function, patients must be evaluated with tone pure audiometry on every 2 weeks or before beginning each section. The treatment must be stopped in case of hearing thresholds becoming higher than 10 dB or in a case of decreasing in speech audiometry of more than 15%. A supportive drug treatment may be necessary until the vertigo control. A pretreatment auditory test is very important. The bone conduction pure tone thresholds average (0.5, 1.0, 2.0, and 3.0 kHz) is considered and repeated every 2 weeks and 2 weeks after treatment. The final audiometric exam is performed up to 12 months after transtympanic protocol initiation.

The success rate in transtympanic injection of gentamicin is about 87% in vertigo control, being a simple and safe procedure with few risks to hearing loss and tympanic membrane perforation [24, 27].

Acknowledgements

The authors wish to thank FAEPA and CAPES.

Conflict of interest

No conflict of interest.

Author details

Maria Stella A. Amaral[1], Henrique F. Pauna[1], Ana Claudia M.B. Reis[2] and Miguel A. Hyppolito[1*]

1 Department of Ophthalmology, Otorhinolaryngology and Head and Neck Surgery, Ribeirão Preto Medical School—University of São Paulo, Ribeirão Preto, São Paulo, Brazil

2 Department of Health Sciences, Ribeirão Preto Medical School—University of São Paulo, Riberão Preto, São Paulo, Brazil

*Address all correspondence to: mahyppo@fmrp.usp.br

References

[1] Gürkov R, Pyykö I, Zou J, Kentala E. What is Menière disease? A contemporary re-evaluation of endolymphatic hydrops. Journal of Neurology. 2016;**263**:71-81

[2] Lopez-Escamez JA, Carey J, Chung W-H, et al. Diagnostic criteria for Mennière's disease. Journal of Vestibular Research. 2015;**25**:1-7

[3] Wright T. Menière's disease. BMJ Clinical Evidence. 2015;**11**:505

[4] Saeed SR. Fortnightly review. Diagnosis and treatment of Ménière's disease. British Medical Journal. 1998;**316**(7128):368-372

[5] Salt AN, Plontke SK. Endolymphatic hydrops: Pathophysiology and experimental models. Otolaryngologic Clinics of North America. 2010;**43**(5):971-983

[6] Soderman AC, Bagger-Sjoback D, Bergenius J, Langius A. Factors influencing quality of life in patients with Meniere's disease, identified by a multidimensional approach. Otology & Neurotology. 2002;**23**(6):941-948

[7] Brookes GB. The pharmacological treatment of Menière's disease. Clinical Otolaryngology and Allied Sciences. 1996;**21**(1):3-11. Review

[8] Maudonnet EN, de Oliveira JA, Rossato M, Hyppolito MA. Gentamicin attenuates gentamicin-induced ototoxicity—Self-protection. Drug and Chemical Toxicology. 2008;**31**(1):11-25

[9] Strose A, Hyppolito MA, Colombari GC, Rossato M, Oliveira JA. Lack of protection against gentamicin ototoxicity by auditory conditioning with noise. Brazilian Journal of Otorhinolaryngology. 2014;**80**(5):390-396

[10] Hellström S, Ödkvist L. Pharmacological labyrinthectomy. Otolaryngologic Clinics of North America. 1994;**27**:307-315

[11] Güneri EA, Çakır A, Mutlu B. Validity and reliability of the diagnostic tests for Ménière's disease. Turkish Archives of Otorhinolaryngology. 2016;**54**:124-130

[12] Hoa M, Friedman RA, Fisher LM, Derebery MJ. Prognostic implications of and audiometric evidence for hearing fluctuation in Meniere's disease. The Laryngoscope. 2015;**125**(12):S1-S12

[13] Carey JP. Ménière's disease. Handbook of Clinical Neurophysiology. Elsevier; Baltimore, United States: 2010. pp. 371-381. DOI: 10.1016/S1567-4231(10)09028-3

[14] Santos PM, Hall RA, Snyder JM, Hughes LF, Dobie RA. Diuretic and diet effect on Menière's disease evaluated by the 1985 Committee on Hearing and Equilibrium guidelines. Otolaryngology and Head and Neck Surgery. 1993;**109**(4):680-689

[15] Nedzelski JM, Schessel DA, Bryce GE, Pheiderer AG. Chemical labyrinthectomy local application of gentamicin for the treatment of unilateral Ménière's disease. The American Journal of Otology. 1992;**13**:18-22

[16] Portmann G. Vertigo: Surgical treatment by opening the saccus endolymphaticus. Archives of Otolaryngology. 1927;**83**:316-319

[17] Beck C. Intratympanic application of gentamicin for treatment of Menière's disease. The Keio Journal of Medicine. 1986;**35**(1):36-41

[18] Cohen-Kerem R, Kisilevsky V, Einarson TR, et al. Intratympanic gentamicin for Ménière's disease: A

meta-analysis. The Laryngoscope. 2004;**114**:2085-2091

[19] Diamond C, O'Connell DA, Hornig JD, et al. Systematic review of intratympanic gentamicin in Ménière's disease. The Journal of Otolaryngology. 2003;**32**:351-361

[20] Stokroos R, Kingma H. Selective vestibular ablation by intratympanic gentamicin in patients with unilateral active Meniere's disease: A prospective, double-blind, placebo-controlled, randomized clinical trial. Acta Oto-Laryngologica. 2004;**124**(2):172-175

[21] Sam G, Chung DW, van der Hoeven R, Verweij S, Becker M. The effect of intratympanic gentamicin for treatment of Ménière's disease on lower frequency hearing. International Journal of Clinical Pharmacy. 2016;**38**(4):780-783. DOI: 10.1007/s11096-016-0295-4

[22] Trune DR, Kempton JB, Kessi M. Aldosterone (mineralocorticoid) equivalent to prednisolone (glucocorticoid) in reversing hearing loss in MRL/MpJ-Fas1pr autoimmune mice. The Laryngoscope. 2000;**110**:1902-1906

[23] Boleas-Aguirre MS, Lin FR, Della Santina CC, Minor LB, Carey JP. Longitudinal results with intratympanic dexamethasone in the treatment of Ménière's disease. Otology & Neurotology. 2008;**29**(1):33-38. DOI: 10.1097/mao.0b013e31815dbafc

[24] Parnes LS, Sun AH, Freeman DJ. Corticosteroid pharmacokinetics in the inner ear fluids: An animal study followed by clinical application. The Laryngoscope. 1999;**109**(7 Pt 2):1-17

[25] Patel M. Intratympanic corticosteroids in Ménière's disease: A mini-review. The Journal of Otolaryngology. 2017;**12**(3):117-124. DOI: 10.1016/j.joto.2017.06.002

[26] Patel M, Agarwal K, Arshad Q, et al. Intratympanic methylprednisolone versus gentamicin in patients with unilateral Meniere's disease: A randomized, double-blind, comparative effectiveness trial. Lancet. 2016;**388**(10061):2753-2762

[27] Chia SH, Gamst AC, Anderson JP, et al. Intratympanic gentamicin therapy for Ménière's disease: A meta-analysis. Otology & Neurotology. 2004;**25**:544-552

Chapter 5

Intratympanic Gentamicin Treatment for Ménière's Disease

Yongchuan Chai and Hongzhe Li

Abstract

Ménière's disease (MD) is an inner-ear disease mostly characterized by frequent spontaneous vertigo and fluctuating sensorineural hearing loss. The main purpose of treatment for MD is to reduce or control the vertigo while maximizing the preservation of hearing. Among the various treatments, one that is effective for refractory MD, intratympanic gentamicin (ITG), relies on its ototoxic property to effectively control the vertigo symptoms of most patients. ITG treatment has relatively few side effects compared with surgically destructive treatments, but it also carries a nonnegligible risk of sensorineural hearing loss. So far, there is no consensus on the dosage and treatment duration of ITG. Most researchers recommend that intratympanic injection of gentamicin is more suitable for patients with unilateral onset and impaired hearing function, who are younger than 65 years old, as well as with frequent and severe vertigo attacks, and ineffective prior conservative treatment. Before an ITG treatment, patients should be adequately informed about the risk of hearing loss, and in order to reduce the risk of deafness, low drug dose and long intervals between injections are recommended. In short, to administer an ITG injection, multiple factors should be comprehensively considered including patient selection, pharmacological mechanism, drug dose, the interval of administration, complications, indications, and contraindications.

Keywords: intratympanic, gentamicin, Ménière's disease, management, aminoglycosides, vertigo, vestibulotoxicity, ototoxicity

1. Introduction

Ménière's disease (MD), also called idiopathic endolymphatic hydrops, is one of the most common causes of dizziness originating in the inner ear. The typical clinical manifestations are frequent spontaneous vertigo, fluctuating sensorineural hearing loss, tinnitus, and/or aural fullness. Vertigo is typically the most debilitating symptom, and control of vertiginous episodes is the primary goal of therapeutic interventions for most patients.

There are numerous available therapeutic options for MD including conservative treatments with dietary modifications, oral medication, procedural treatments with intratympanic therapies, and surgical treatments. A failure of conservative therapy often introduces the need for a more aggressive therapy on the treatment algorithm.

Surgical intervention or intratympanic aminoglycosides can be used in patients with intractable vertigo, which, ideally, should control the vertigo while preserving the hearing level and balance. The side effects of aminoglycosides are well-know. The risks of vestibular and cochlear toxicity are mainly related to types of aminoglycosides, route of administration, duration of the therapy, total or cumulative dose, individual susceptibility, renal function, patient's age, etc.

In 1948, Fowler [1] first used systemic streptomycin to treat vertigo attacks in patients with intractable MD. The results showed that vertigo attacks could be well controlled, but treatment carried the risks of bilateral vestibulopathy, nephrotoxicity, and unpredictable results. In 1957, Schuknekt [2] may have been the first to use intratympanic streptomycin to alleviate vertigo attacks in patients with unilateral intractable MD, and it was firstly named "chemical labyrinthectomy". Intratympanic gentamicin (ITG) for the treatment of severe vertigo was reported by Lange [3]. The initial approach was complete vestibular ablation to control the vertigo. However, with this approach, the hearing was at a greater risk. Over the past decades, the pharmacological mechanisms of aminoglycosides have been progressively studied in depth and clinical trials have been extensively developed.

At present, intratympanic injection of gentamicin is probably the most effective non-surgical treatment to eradicate vertigo in MD and is gradually gaining popularity in the worldwide. Compared with the treatment regimen decades ago, several modifications for ITG treatment have emerged regarding the concentration of the gentamicin solution, the frequency of injections, and the method of delivery. In this chapter, the history, background, and progression of ITG treatment for MD are discussed, as well as the basic science, therapeutic method, treatment efficacy, indications, contraindications, and complications.

2. History of intratympanic gentamicin

Aminoglycosides are highly potent, broad-spectrum antibiotics and are widely used by various routes of injection to treat serious infections caused by Gram-negative bacteria (e.g., *Pseudomonas aeruginosa*, *Proteus* species, *Escherichia coli*, *Klebsiella-Enterobacter-Serratia* species, and *Citrobacter* species), and are sometimes used as an adjuvant treatment for infections caused by Gram-positive bacteria (e.g., *Staphylococcus* species). The basic chemical structure required for both potency and the spectrum of antimicrobial activity of aminoglycosides is that of one, or several, aminated sugars joined in glycosidic linkages to a dibasic cyclitol. Aminoglycosides act primarily by impairing bacterial protein synthesis through binding to prokaryotic ribosomes [4].

Streptomycin, which was discovered in 1944, is the first aminoglycoside antibiotic in human history and was thereafter marked by the successive introduction of a series of milestone compounds (kanamycin discovered in 1957, gentamicin in 1963, and neomycin in 1970s) which definitively established the usefulness of this class of antibiotics for the treatment of Gram-negative bacillary infections. From the 1960s to 1970s, aminoglycosides were widely used, but due to their serious ototoxicity and nephrotoxicity, their systemic application was limited, and they were gradually fading out of the ranks of first-line drugs. At the beginning, the most common side effect of streptomycin used by intravenous injection was temporary imbalance without vertigo or nystagmus. Higher systemic doses increased the chance of permanent imbalance and, occasionally, deafness. These early observations led to animal and cadaver studies which confirmed the vestibulotoxic and cochleotoxic effects of high-dose streptomycin.

Based on its vestibulotoxicity, streptomycin foremost unveiled its potential in the treatment of vestibular diseases. In 1948, about 4 years after streptomycin was discovered, Fowler [1] first used systemic streptomycin to treat vertigo attacks in patients with intractable MD which was refractory to traditional medical treatment. He and others used between 2 and 4 g of intramuscular streptomycin per day in patients with unilateral or bilateral MD, typically until onset of severe imbalance, and reported that vertigo attacks could be well controlled without loss of hearing. Often, and especially with higher dosing, vertigo control was accompanied with the troubling symptoms of permanent, severe imbalance, and oscillopsia.

In 1957, Schuknecht [2] may have been the first to use intratympanic streptomycin to alleviate vertigo attacks in patients with unilateral MD that was uncontrolled by traditional medical management. He conceived of this idea after noting that intratympanic formalin will readily pass into the inner ear and prevented postmortem degeneration of the inner ear membranous structures in patients. He correctly theorized that streptomycin could also pass into the inner ear and devised a cat animal model that demonstrated clinical and pathologic vestibulotoxicity with intratympanic streptomycin. Based on these results, he devised a clinical trial of intratympanic streptomycin administration to patients with uncontrolled unilateral MD. He administered variable amounts of streptomycin (between 0.125 and 0.5 g), either hourly or over 4 hours, over a variable amount of days. The first group of three patients who received 1 or 2 days of treatment achieved only brief control of their vertigo, but did not lose any hearing. Subsequently, an additional group of five patients received streptomycin for 3 days or longer. These patients had permanent resolution of their vertigo episodes, but at the cost of deafening the ear. Schuknekt coined the term "chemical labyrinthectomy" to describe this phenomenon. He concluded that intratympanic streptomycin at the therapeutic dosage failed to preserve hearing, and should only be considered for patients who are not good surgical candidates, but would otherwise be proper candidates for inner ear ablation [2].

With the administration of intratympanic aminoglycosides, chemical ablation of the inner ear via systemic administration of aminoglycosides fell into disfavor due to the side effects of bilateral vestibulopathy, nephrotoxicity, and unpredictable results. However, choosing which kind of aminoglycoside for intratympanic injection has gradually changed. In 1977, Lange [3] appears to be the first to have used IT administration of gentamicin. He reported about 55 patients suffering from severe unilateral MD, seen over a period of 3–10 years. Patients were treated with intratympanic administration of streptomycin or better, gentamicin. The medication was given using a plastic tube inserted behind the annulus within the transmeatal approach, and 0.1 ml gentamicin (earlier streptomycin) was instilled every 5 hours until the first signs of inner ear reaction (nystagmus or vertigo) appeared. In 90% of the cases, vertiginous attacks ceased after therapy, and hearing was preserved in 76%.

Entering the 1990s, intratympanic gentamicin had gained widespread popularity in the treatment of MD. Compared with streptomycin, ITG for treatment of MD provided equivalently excellent vertigo control while showing a lower incidence of hearing loss in early clinical data. Gentamicin gained popularity over streptomycin and gradually came to be the drug of choice for chemical ablation of inner ear.

In 1993, Nedzelski et al. [5] studied 50 patients with unilateral MD by treatment of microcatheter administration of streptomycin over a 5 h treatment, 4 treatments within 48 hours, and the rate of vertigo control was up to 96%; only 24% of his patients experienced various degrees of hearing loss. Although streptomycin was being used in the study, he advocated for using gentamicin instead for its theoretical reduction of cochleotoxicity.

Beck and Schmidt [6] reported on their 10 years of experience with intratympanally applied streptomycin and gentamicin in the therapy of MD. They theorized that the dosage might be a critical factor for hearing preservation with vertigo control. Aminoglycosides could be titrated to impede the secretory epithelium of the vestibular apparatus without destroying the sensory cells, thus achieving vertigo control while maintaining caloric response, that is, vestibulo-ocular reflex. More importantly, risk of deafness could potentially be eliminated. By reducing the dosage delivered and titrating, they were able to achieve excellent rates of vertigo control (92%) while also achieving respectable hearing preservation rates (15% hearing loss with no cases of deafness).

During the same era, around the early 1990s, two schools of thought emerged in an effort to standardize ITG treatment, dubbed the "shotgun" approach, and the "low-dose" approach. The shotgun approach, championed by Nedzelski and others [5], was characterized by daily IT injections to a fixed endpoint or to a clinical threshold that heralded damage to the inner ear. Proponents of this approach attempted to achieve adequate vestibular ablation for long-term vertigo control. The low-dose approach, championed by Magnusson and others [7], was characterized by weekly IT injections, also to a fixed endpoint or to clinical effect. Proponents of this approach tried to achieve vertigo control while minimizing damage to hearing and potentially preserving the caloric response as well.

Today, intratympanic injection of gentamicin is probably the most effective non-surgical treatment to eradicate vertigo in MD. Yet, it is an ablative method that carries a non-negligible risk of hearing loss. Currently, gentamicin is usually instilled via IT injection or through a tympanostomy tube to the round window niche. These injections are repeated over a variable amount of time, typically between daily to weekly injections, until a clinical endpoint is achieved or until there is a decline in hearing. No consensus has been reached so far on the overall dosage, dosing methods, timing of delivery, treatment duration, clinical endpoint of therapy, or concentration of gentamicin. Both clinical evidence and basic science models should be further studied to scientifically elicit the most effective and safe regimen.

3. Mechanism of action

Aminoglycoside antibiotics have a well-documented history of cochleotoxic and vestibulotoxic effects. Administration of intratympanic aminoglycoside antibiotics to patients with MD is based on the notion that the patient's vestibular symptoms are due to the damaged and distorted vestibular signals emanating from their ear and that they are better off with no signal than with a damaged and distorted signal. The objective of ITG is to weaken vestibular signals in the Ménière's ear to the point at which they are no longer strong enough to generate a vertigo attack. Ideally, aminoglycosides would act to reduce vestibular function, and thus alleviate the patient's symptoms of vertigo, while preserving hearing. The degree to which a drug is cochleotoxic or vestibulotoxic differs among aminoglycosides. Gentamicin and streptomycin, for instance, are reported to be more vestibulotoxic. Other aminoglycosides, such as amikacin, are considered to be relatively more cochleotoxic and thus are not used transtympanically. The best evidence for this is the simple clinical observation that patients undergoing systemic gentamicin or streptomycin therapy experience vestibulopathy much more commonly than hearing loss. This feature has been used by otologists to control the vestibular symptoms of MD, initially provided through systemic delivery by Fowler [1] and subsequently through IT injections by Schuknecht [2, 8]. Use of streptomycin has been largely replaced by gentamicin which is thought to be more selectively vestibulotoxic and better able to preserve residual hearing in patients with unilateral MD refractory to medical management [9, 10].

Within the bony labyrinth, several studies have investigated the trafficking and distribution of aminoglycosides, finding different patterns of distribution dependent upon the dose, duration, and route of administration. IT-injected aminoglycosides appear to gain access to the inner ear via the oval window and the round window [11, 12], and uptake either by passive diffusion or by endocytosis [13, 14]. Salt et al. recently quantified diffusion of gentamicin through the oval (35%)

versus the round window (57%) [12, 15]. Access to these membranous structures is however uncertain, partly due to their variable permeability in individuals, resulting in unpredictable drug exposure of the inner ear [16–18]. Similar mechanisms of cellular trafficking (active diffusion and endocytosis) have been proposed in the transport of aminoglycosides into cells of the inner ear [19].

Once the drug crosses the oval window and the round window, the situation becomes more complex and the precise mechanism by which aminoglycosides exert their toxic effects on hair cells is unknown, to date. Previous animal studies showed that in the cochlea, sensory hair cells, the spiral ligament including the stria vascularis, and spiral ganglion cells had a very early uptake of gentamicin. Similarly, hair cells, dark cells, and vestibular ganglion cells are the primary targets in the vestibular system. This may demonstrate that gentamicin most likely diffuses across the inner ear membranes, readily achieving concentrations within the scala vestibuli, cochlear duct, and vestibule and then exerts its cellular toxicity.

Multiple mechanisms, including disruption of calcium-dependent cytokine production resulting in the damage to hair cell membrane integrity, increased superoxide production, hair cell transduction blockage, glutamate decarboxylase inhibition, ornithine decarboxylase inhibition, and free radical damage, all have been developed to explain aminoglycosides' direct toxicity to hair cells [10, 20, 21]. While most cells of the inner ear demonstrate aminoglycoside penetration, several studies have identified preferential loss of the hair cells at the basal turn of the cochlea over the apical hair cells and vestibular type I hair cells over their type II counterparts [22–26]. Direct damage to the spiral ganglion has also been observed [27] and histologic studies in rhesus monkeys suggest relative sparing of the maculae [28].

In parallel to previous findings, several studies have demonstrated that direct application of gentamicin into the vestibular labyrinth also causes greater loss of type I versus type II vestibular hair cells [29, 30]. Recently, Lyford-Pike et al. [26] used the animal model, chinchilla, to provide the evidence that the selective loss of type I hair cells assuredly occurred because these cells preferentially accumulate gentamicin acutely after intratympanic administration. Type II hair cells and supporting cells concentrate substantially less gentamicin. These results might theoretically ameliorate the more profound symptom of vertigo (driven by type I hair cells) while preserving cochlear function.

Aminoglycosides may also act to inhibit production of endolymph, restoring the balance between endolymphatic and perilymphatic pressure. This would also act to alleviate all symptoms of endolymphatic hydrops. Additionally, aminoglycosides are theorized to cause selective damage to the cells of the cochlear stria vascularis and planum semilunatum in the cristae ampullae of the semicircular canals, which are involved in ionic regulation and endolymph production [31]. It is also known that gentamicin utilizes the cellular machinery of endolymph production to traffic into the inner ear after systemic administration [32]. The theory that vestibular dark cells and, thus, endolymphatic flow, are the targets by which aminoglycosides alleviate vertigo is of significant clinical interest because it suggests that it is not necessarily important to ablate the vestibule to achieve vertigo control in MD. This idea can explain why patients with intact caloric responses can still achieve significant vertigo control after intratympanic aminoglycoside administration.

In conclusion, direct toxicity to vestibular hair cells and direct toxicity to the endolymph producing apparatus might be the two major mechanisms of action by ITG. Most importantly, gentamicin has been proved to be more vestibulotoxic than cochleotoxic in humans. The inner ear toxicity of gentamicin might follow an order. Secretory dark cells of the vestibule might be the first to be damaged, followed by the vestibular neuroepithelium and the afferent vestibular fibers, and finally, the hair cells of the organ of Corti are destroyed [33, 34].

4. Therapeutic method and treatment efficacy

Ménière's disease is manifested by episodic vertigo, tinnitus, aural fullness, and fluctuating hearing loss. The treatment of patients with MD is usually directed at the most disabling symptom, which is the debilitating vertigo. MD treatment protocols typically measure vertigo control according to AAO-HNS Committee on Hearing and Equilibrium guidelines for grading vertigo severity [35]. Often, clinical trials also attempt to assess other disease sequelae such as hearing loss, tinnitus, and aural fullness.

As a well-known relapsing-remitting disease, it is rather difficult to accurately evaluate the efficacy of ITG in treatment of MD. Firstly, the natural history of remission and exacerbation of symptoms make evaluation of the effectiveness of treatment remarkably difficult. Commonly, vertigo attacks can improve without treatment of any kind as periods of remission are not uncommon. Thus, a clinical trial without controls will not account for this finding. Another difficulty is that clinical researchers attempt to show hearing preservation with IT gentamicin protocol, but hearing tends to worsen over time in MD regardless of treatment. Finally, the variable nature of MD with fluctuation in levels of hearing and even frequency and severity of vertigo can make clinical trials difficult.

To date, there have only been a few interventional randomized controlled trials investigating the true efficacy of ITG in the treatment of MD. In 2004, the first prospective, double-blind, randomized clinical trial of intratympanic gentamicin versus intratympanic buffer solution (placebo) in patients with active MD was reported by Stokroos et al. [36]. They performed ITG injections with buffered gentamicin (30 mg/ml) every 6 weeks until the vertigo complaints disappeared (12 patients received gentamicin versus 10 for placebo), outcome measures included the number of vertiginous spells, degree of sensorineural hearing loss, labyrinthine function, and labyrinthine asymmetry. Compared to the placebo group, topical gentamicin provided a significant improvement in the number of vertiginous attacks per year at follow up which varied between 6 and 28 months. There was no statistically significant change in hearing or other outcomes in two groups. However, hearing had a tendency to deteriorate in the placebo-treated patients, due to the natural course of the disease, which suggests that early treatment with topical gentamicin may preserve residual sensorineural hearing in active MD.

In 2008, Postema et al. [37] reported another prospective, double-blind, randomized, placebo-controlled trial associated with ITG therapy for control of vertigo in unilateral MD. They used weekly injections of 0.4 ml of gentamicin (30 mg/ml). A total of 4 injections were given through a ventilation tube (16 patients received gentamicin and 12 received a placebo). The results showed that gentamicin treatment resulted in a significant reduction of the score for vertigo complaints (including vertigo severity) and the score for perceived aural fullness. They also noted that a small increase in hearing loss (average of losses at 0.5, 1, 2, and 4 kHz: 8 dB HL) was measured in the gentamicin group.

In 2016, Patel et al. [38] performed a randomized, double-blind, comparative effectiveness trial of intratympanic methylprednisolone (n = 30) versus gentamicin (n = 30) in patients with refractory unilateral MD. Patients were randomly assigned (1:1) to two intratympanic methylprednisolone (62.5 mg/ml) or gentamicin (40 mg/ml) injections given 2 weeks apart, and were followed up for 2 years. In the methylprednisolone group, complete vertigo control (Class A) was achieved in 21/30 patients

(70%) compared to 25/30 (83.3%) in the gentamicin group. After methylprednisolone, 22 patients (78.5%) experienced an improved functional level score and 8 patients (28.7%) better pure-tone hearing and speech discrimination. There were also reductions for tinnitus, dizziness, and aural fullness. Fifteen patients (50%) required further courses of methylprednisolone. Two patients were deemed treatment failures and were assigned ITG treatment. The study showed no significant difference between the methylprednisolone and gentamicin for the control of vertigo, total number of injections, number of patients with relapsing vertigo, or the amount of pain from injection but better speech discrimination after methylprednisolone.

Based on the above prospective, double-blind, randomized controlled clinical trials, intratympanic gentamicin, as a medically ablative method, seems to be the most effective non-surgical treatment to eradicate vertigo in intractable MD, but with a potential risk of hearing loss. However, there is no consensus on the treatment protocol of ITG, especially for the concentration of gentamicin, dosage in each application, number of injection, and the time interval between two doses.

In the over 40 years of clinical trials in the treatment of MD by ITG, the majority are case series without controls, mainly because of the significant difficulties in conducting the randomized controlled clinical trials or case/control trials [33]. In earlier studies, the highest rate of vertigo control was reported with daily injections or multiple titrations. On the other hand, considerable hearing loss was experienced in several studies. Moller et al. [39] treated 15 patients with disabling MD with daily injections for periods ranging from 3 to 11 days. They achieved 93.4% of vertigo control, but also 33.4% of hearing loss. They reported that none of the patients were responsive to caloric stimulation. Laitakari [40] reported 90% of vertigo control and 45% of hearing loss in 20 patients who had daily ITG for a minimum of 3 consecutive days. Parnes and Riddell [41] reported 41.7% worsening of the hearing in their group of patients who received three daily injections within 4 days. Murofushi et al. [42], using several daily injections, reported hearing loss in 30% of cases. Corsten et al. [43] reported 81% vertigo control but 57% hearing loss in patients (n = 21) who had gentamicin instillation 3 times a day for 4 consecutive days. Kaplan et al. [44] reviewed the 10-year long-term results of 114 patients treated with gentamicin instillation 3 times a day for 4 consecutive days. They achieved 93.4% of vertigo control and 25.6% of hearing loss.

In the early 2000s, regarding patients with hearing deterioration and even those becoming deaf, there was a discussion about reducing the gentamicin dose or performing the application at longer intervals. Daily titration methods were abandoned. Transtympanic gentamicin therapy was modified to weekly or monthly intervals as "needed" or "on demand" to reduce the symptoms of MD, aiming to maintain cochlear as well as vestibular function. Harner et al. [45] reported a very high rate of vertigo control with preservation of hearing in 43 patients. There were no patients with changes in cochlear function and ablation of the labyrinth. All patients received one injection, and half of them received a repeat injection 1 month after therapy. Minor [46] used gentamicin on weekly intervals until the development of spontaneous nystagmus, head-shaking nystagmus, or head thrust sign. Vertigo was controlled in 91% of the patients, and profound hearing loss only occurred in 1 patient. Atlas and Parnes [47] reviewed the outcomes of 83 patients who received weekly injections. They reported hearing loss in 17% of the patients, with vertigo control in 84%. Martin and Perez [48] reported vertigo control in 83.1% of the patients and hearing loss in 15.5% of them after gentamicin at weekly intervals. De Beer et al. [49] reported 15.8% with hearing loss and 80.7% with vertigo control after, between 1 and 10, intratympanic injections at a minimum interval of 27 days. Casani et al. [50] reported 12% hearing loss after a maximum of 2 injections of gentamicin and 81% vertigo control.

Most recently, Vlastarakos et al. [51] published a systematic review looking at sustained-release delivery of IT gentamicin (dynamic-release versus sustained-release vehicles). Dynamic release (microcatheter at the round window) was found to provide satisfactory vertigo control in 89.3% (70.9% reporting complete control). Sustained-release preparations (gentamicin-soaked wick/pledget) provided 82.2% satisfactory control in the pool of patients (75% with complete control). In patients receiving sustained-release preparations, complete hearing loss was reported in 31.1% patients with another 23.3% of patients experiencing partial hearing loss. This adverse change in hearing was unacceptably high, reinforcing the suggestion of using a sustained-release vehicle only in patients who had failed IT gentamicin injections previously or those without serviceable hearing.

Commonly, intratympanic injection under otoscope or microscope is a simple and recommendable technique. The desired amount of gentamicin is injected over the round window through the posterosuperior quadrant of the tympanic membrane. There are two common doses of gentamicin for injection. The standard intravenous preparation of gentamicin is 40 mg/ml, which can be buffered with 8.4% sodium bicarbonate so that discomfort on injection is reduced. A total of 1.5 ml of gentamicin mixed with 0.5 ml of sodium bicarbonate at these concentrations will produce a final concentration of 26.6 mg/ml gentamicin. Approximately 0.3–0.5 ml of solution is usually adequate to bathe the round window in solution. Typically, patients will remain lying flat with the injected ear up for 10 min to 1 h. This procedure is generally well tolerated by patients, who should be told to expect brief pain on injection, followed by possible vertigo or disequilibrium. Warming the medication can help in this regard (preventing a cold caloric response).

Based on the combination of current clinical practice, basic science models, and results from clinical trials, low drug dose and long interval between injections, mainly in order to reduce the risk of deafness, are reasonably encouraged. The low dose method involves using 1–2 injections of gentamicin and waiting a month or 2 weeks between injections. The rate of vertigo control may be up to 80–90%, with no significant side effects. The second injection is given only if there has been a vertigo spell 2 weeks prior. In other words, instead of titrating to the onset of damage to the vestibular system, the criterion is a positive effect on the disease. Occasionally, a third dose is given.

In short, whatever technique is used, the goal is to apply gentamicin to the round window in sufficient concentration and over a sufficient amount of time that it achieves a therapeutic effect while avoiding both local and systemic side effects, especially hearing loss.

5. Indications and contraindications

Not all patients with MD can be treated with ITG. Based on the international consensus on treatment of MD obtained from the IFOS meeting 2017 [52], MD should be treated with a step-by-step therapy. The first line of treatment includes the medical conservative treatment, such as dietary modification and oral medicine. After this line of treatment, 80% of patients with MD are cured or in remission. When the vertigo of MD fails to be controlled by the first-line treatment for more than 6 months, it will be regarded as intractable MD. Then the second line is the IT injections, mainly IT steroids as a conservative treatment and ITG in the case of IT steroid failure, and preferentially in patients with hearing impairment. After the second line treatment, 90–95% of the total patients are cured or in remission. The third line is the surgical, either conservative or destructive, treatment. For unilateral intractable MD with serviceable hearing (i.e., speech reception threshold better than 50 dB HL and speech discrimination score of more than 50%) in the treated ear, treatment protocol with an injection repetition not shorter than 1 week between adjacent injections or one with injections on a monthly basis as "needed" is preferred. These methods provide the same level of vertigo control yet offer better preservation of hearing functions [33].

The best indication for ITG treatment appears to be the control of vertigo in profound hearing loss or non-serviceable ears, in which speech reception threshold is worse than 50 dB HL and speech discrimination score less than 50% [53, 54]. Under these scenarios, there is no need to consider the risk of deafness, and titration methods or multiple injections on a daily basis are preferred, since these methods have significantly elevated incidence of hearing loss [33]. Transmastoid labyrinthectomy has traditionally been offered for non-serviceable ears in patients with MD. This method has been the gold standard, and it is very effective in eradication of vertigo in more than 94% of patients. In comparison, ITG therapy provides a minimally invasive ambulatory substitute with low morbidity and fewer side-effects, which is also very cost effective to manage vertigo in these MD patients with non-serviceable ears [53].

Another important indicator is the control of vertigo in patients who have failed endolymphatic sac surgery. Marzo and Leonetti [55] have shown the effectiveness of ITG therapy for patients who have failed endolymphatic sac surgery, thus reducing the need for vestibular neurectomy in those with intractable disease.

To be allergic and hypersensitive to aminoglycosides are two absolute contraindications for ITG. It is worth noting that patients who carried the mitochondrial mutation of the gene MT-RNR1 (mitochondrially encoded 12S ribosomal RNA) are hypersensitive to aminoglycosides. A single injection of aminoglycosides results in complete and definitive deafness in subjects with this mutation [56]. A systematic genetic screening of MD patients is highly recommended to prevent the occurrence of bilateral deafness. The treatment is intended for the abolition of vestibular function; thus, administration of gentamicin must be done carefully in the elderly, who have difficulty attaining vestibular compensation, in patients with complications, or in those with bilateral MD. Taking also into consideration the fact that individual's drug sensitivity depends on their genetic background, investigation of appropriate drug levels according to evidence-based medicine remains a future task.

6. Complications

The complications of ITG treatment are primarily bi-fold: one is the risk caused by drug toxicity of gentamicin, the other is the risk caused by intratympanic injection. Undoubtedly, the main risk of ITG treatment for vertigo is the sensorineural hearing loss and associated prolonged disequilibrium and ataxia, which are common complaints after this treatment. Less common side effects include local hemorrhage, allergic response and tympanic membrane perforation (especially in an irradiated or otherwise damaged tympanic membrane), local discomfort, inflammation, otitis media or externa, and transient vertigo caused by a caloric reflex effect from the instilled fluid [38, 57]. It is also critical to educate all patients who are given intratympanic aminoglycosides that bilateral permanent hearing loss is possible, even from one single unilateral injection.

7. Conclusions

Intratympanic injection of gentamicin is probably the most effective non-surgical treatment to eradicate vertigo in MD. But it is also an ablative method that carries a non-negligible risk of hearing loss. Gentamicin has been proved to be more vestibulotoxic than cochleotoxic; direct toxicity to vestibular hair cells and direct toxicity to the endolymph producing apparatus might be the two major mechanisms of action. To date, no consensus has been reached on the dosage, dosing methods, timing of delivery, treatment duration, clinical endpoint of therapy, and concentration of gentamicin. However, based on the combination of current clinical practice, basic science models, and results from clinical trials, low drug dose and long intervals between injections are reasonably recommended. The application of gentamicin-induced vestibular ablation has minimized the number of more invasive procedures such as unilateral labyrinthectomy and vestibular neurectomy. In comparison with surgery, the vertigo control is comparable, the overall cost is reduced, and complications are limited. ITG in treating intractable MD has gradually become a prevalent therapy during the past decades. However, to administer ITG treatment, multiple factors should be comprehensively considered including patient selection, pharmacological mechanism, drug dose, the interval of administration, complications, indications, and contraindications.

Acknowledgements

The authors thank Alisa Hetrick for her comments on an earlier version of the article.

Conflict of interest

The authors declare no competing financial interest.

Author details

Yongchuan Chai[1,2,3,4,5] and Hongzhe Li[1,2,6]*

1 Research Service, VA Loma Linda Healthcare System, Loma Linda, CA, United States

2 Loma Linda University School of Medicine, Loma Linda, CA, United States

3 Department of Otorhinolaryngology—Head and Neck Surgery, Shanghai Ninth People's Hospital, Shanghai Jiao Tong University School of Medicine, Shanghai, China

4 Ear Institute, Shanghai Jiao Tong University School of Medicine, Shanghai, China

5 Shanghai Key Laboratory of Translational Medicine on Ear and Nose Diseases, Shanghai, China

6 Department of Otolaryngology—Head and Neck Surgery, Loma Linda University School of Medicine, Loma Linda, CA, United States

*Address all correspondence to: hongzhe.li@va.gov; hongzhe@gmail.com

References

[1] Fowler EP Jr. Streptomycin treatment of vertigo. Transactions of the American Academy of Ophthalmology and Otolaryngology. 1948;**52**:293-301

[2] Schuknecht HF. Ablation therapy in the management of Meniere's disease. Acta Oto-Laryngologica. Supplementum. 1957;**132**:1-42

[3] Lange G. The intratympanic treatment of Meniere's disease with ototoxic antibiotics. A follow-up study of 55 cases (author's transl). Laryngologie, Rhinologie, Otologie. 1977;**56**:409-414

[4] Mingeot-Leclercq MP, Glupczynski Y, Tulkens PM. Aminoglycosides: Activity and resistance. Antimicrobial Agents and Chemotherapy. 1999;**43**:727-737

[5] Nedzelski JM, Chiong CM, Fradet G, Schessel DA, Bryce GE, Pfleiderer AG. Intratympanic gentamicin instillation as treatment of unilateral Meniere's disease: Update of an ongoing study. The American Journal of Otology. 1993;**14**:278-282

[6] Beck C, Schmidt CL. 10 years of experience with intratympanally applied streptomycin (gentamycin) in the therapy of Morbus Meniere. Archives of Oto-Rhino-Laryngology. 1978;**221**:149-152

[7] Magnusson M, Padoan S. Delayed onset of ototoxic effects of gentamicin in treatment of Meniere's disease. Rationale for extremely low dose therapy. Acta Oto-Laryngologica. 1991;**111**:671-676

[8] Schuknecht HF. Ablation therapy for the relief of Meniere's disease. Laryngoscope. 1956;**66**:859-870

[9] Webster JC, McGee TM, Carroll R, Benitez JT, Williams ML. Ototoxicity of gentamicin. Histopathologic and functional results in the cat. Transactions of the American Academy of Ophthalmology and Otolaryngology. 1970;**74**:1155-1165

[10] Rudnick MD, Ginsberg IA, Huber PS. Aminoglycoside ototoxicity following middle ear injection. The Annals of Otology, Rhinology and Laryngology. Supplement. 1980;**89**:i-iii, 1-28

[11] Smith BM, Myers MG. The penetration of gentamicin and neomycin into perilymph across the round window membrane. Otolaryngology—Head and Neck Surgery. 1979;**87**:888-891

[12] Salt AN, Hartsock JJ, Gill RM, King E, Kraus FB, Plontke SK. Perilymph pharmacokinetics of locally-applied gentamicin in the guinea pig. Hearing Research. 2016;**342**:101-111

[13] Goycoolea MV. Clinical aspects of round window membrane permeability under normal and pathological conditions. Acta Oto-Laryngologica. 2001;**121**:437-447

[14] Becvarovski Z, Bojrab DI, Michaelides EM, Kartush JM, Zappia JJ, LaRouere MJ. Round window gentamicin absorption: An in vivo human model. The Laryngoscope. 2002;**112**:1610-1613

[15] Salt AN, Ma Y. Quantification of solute entry into cochlear perilymph through the round window membrane. Hearing Research. 2001;**154**:88-97

[16] Silverstein H, Rowan PT, Olds MJ, Rosenberg SI. Inner ear perfusion and the role of round window patency. The American Journal of Otology. 1997;**18**:586-589

[17] Yoshioka M, Naganawa S, Sone M, Nakata S, Teranishi M,

Nakashima T. Individual differences in the permeability of the round window: Evaluating the movement of intratympanic gadolinium into the inner ear. Otology and Neurotology. 2009;**30**:645-648

[18] Alzamil KS, Linthicum FH Jr. Extraneous round window membranes and plugs: Possible effect on intratympanic therapy. The Annals of Otology, Rhinology, and Laryngology. 2000;**109**:30-32

[19] Carey J. Intratympanic gentamicin for the treatment of Meniere's disease and other forms of peripheral vertigo. Otolaryngologic Clinics of North America. 2004;**37**:1075-1090

[20] Williams SE, Zenner HP, Schacht J. Three molecular steps of aminoglycoside ototoxicity demonstrated in outer hair cells. Hearing Research. 1987;**30**:11-18

[21] Schacht J. Biochemical basis of aminoglycoside ototoxicity. Otolaryngologic Clinics of North America. 1993;**26**:845-856

[22] Wersall J, Lundquist PG, Bjorkroth B. Ototoxicity of gentamicin. The Journal of Infectious Diseases. 1969;**119**:410-416

[23] Lindeman HH. Regional differences in sensitivity of the vestibular sensory epithelia to ototoxic antibiotics. Acta Oto-Laryngologica. 1969;**67**:177-189

[24] de Groot JC, Meeuwsen F, Ruizendaal WE, Veldman JE. Ultrastructural localization of gentamicin in the cochlea. Hearing Research. 1990;**50**:35-42

[25] Tsuji K, Velazquez-Villasenor L, Rauch SD, Glynn RJ, Wall C, Merchant SN. Temporal bone studies of the human peripheral vestibular system. Aminoglycoside ototoxicity. The Annals of Otology, Rhinology and Laryngology Supplement. 2000;**181**:20-25

[26] Lyford-Pike S, Vogelheim C, Chu E, Della Santina CC, Carey JP. Gentamicin is primarily localized in vestibular type I hair cells after intratympanic administration. Journal of the Association for Research in Otolaryngology: JARO. 2007;**8**:497-508

[27] Bae WY, Kim LS, Hur DY, Jeong SW, Kim JR. Secondary apoptosis of spiral ganglion cells induced by aminoglycoside: Fas–Fas ligand signaling pathway. The Laryngoscope. 2008;**118**:1659-1668

[28] Sun DQ, Lehar M, Dai C, Swarthout L, Lauer AM, Carey JP, et al. Histopathologic changes of the inner ear in Rhesus monkeys after intratympanic gentamicin injection and vestibular prosthesis electrode array implantation. Journal of the Association for Research in Otolaryngology: JARO. 2015;**16**:373-387

[29] Lopez I, Honrubia V, Lee SC, Schoeman G, Beykirch K. Quantification of the process of hair cell loss and recovery in the chinchilla crista ampullaris after gentamicin treatment. International Journal of Developmental Neuroscience. 1997;**15**:447-461

[30] Hirvonen TP, Minor LB, Hullar TE, Carey JP. Effects of intratympanic gentamicin on vestibular afferents and hair cells in the chinchilla. Journal of Neurophysiology. 2005;**93**:643-655

[31] Atlas J, Parnes LS. Intratympanic gentamicin for intractable Meniere's disease: 5-year follow-up. The Journal of Otolaryngology. 2003;**32**:288-293

[32] Li H, Steyger PS. Systemic aminoglycosides are trafficked via endolymph into cochlear hair cells. Scientific Reports. 2011;**1**:159

[33] Yetiser S. Intratympanic gentamicin for intractable Meniere's disease—A review and analysis of audiovestibular impact. International Archives of Otorhinolaryngology. 2018;**22**:190-194

[34] Sultemeier DR, Hoffman LF. Partial aminoglycoside lesions in vestibular epithelia reveal broad sensory dysfunction associated with modest hair cell loss and afferent calyx retraction. Frontiers in Cellular Neuroscience. 2017;**11**:331

[35] Monsell EM. New and revised reporting guidelines from the committee on hearing and equilibrium. Otolaryngology—Head and Neck Surgery. 1995;**113**:176-178

[36] Stokroos R, Kingma H. Selective vestibular ablation by intratympanic gentamicin in patients with unilateral active Meniere's disease: A prospective, double-blind, placebo-controlled, randomized clinical trial. Acta Oto-Laryngologica. 2004;**124**:172-175

[37] Postema RJ, Kingma CM, Wit HP, Albers FW, Van Der Laan BF. Intratympanic gentamicin therapy for control of vertigo in unilateral Menire's disease: A prospective, double-blind, randomized, placebo-controlled trial. Acta Oto-Laryngologica. 2008;**128**:876-880

[38] Patel M, Agarwal K, Arshad Q, Hariri M, Rea P, Seemungal BM, et al. Intratympanic methylprednisolone versus gentamicin in patients with unilateral Meniere's disease: A randomized, double-blind, comparative effectiveness trial. Lancet. 2016;**388**:2753-2762

[39] Moller C, Odkvist LM, Thell J, Larsby B, Hyden D. Vestibular and audiologic functions in gentamicin-treated Meniere's disease. The American Journal of Otology. 1988;**9**:383-391

[40] Laitakari K. Intratympanic gentamycin in severe Meniere's disease. Clinical Otolaryngology and Allied Sciences. 1990;**15**:545-548

[41] Parnes LS, Riddell D. Irritative spontaneous nystagmus following intratympanic gentamicin for Meniere's disease. The Laryngoscope. 1993;**103**:745-749

[42] Murofushi T, Halmagyi GM, Yavor RA. Intratympanic gentamicin in Meniere's disease: Results of therapy. The American Journal of Otology. 1997;**18**:52-57

[43] Corsten M, Marsan J, Schramm D, Robichaud J. Treatment of intractable Meniere's disease with intratympanic gentamicin: Review of the University of Ottawa experience. The Journal of Otolaryngology. 1997;**26**:361-364

[44] Kaplan DM, Nedzelski JM, Al-Abidi A, Chen JM, Shipp DB. Hearing loss following intratympanic instillation of gentamicin for the treatment of unilateral Meniere's disease. The Journal of Otolaryngology. 2002;**31**:106-111

[45] Harner SG, Kasperbauer JL, Facer GW, Beatty CW. Transtympanic gentamicin for Meniere's syndrome. The Laryngoscope. 1998;**108**:1446-1449

[46] Minor LB. Intratympanic gentamicin for control of vertigo in Meniere's disease: Vestibular signs that specify completion of therapy. The American Journal of Otology. 1999;**20**:209-219

[47] Atlas JT, Parnes LS. Intratympanic gentamicin titration therapy for intractable Meniere's disease. The American Journal of Otology. 1999;**20**:357-363

[48] Martin E, Perez N. Hearing loss after intratympanic gentamicin therapy for unilateral Meniere's disease. Otology and Neurotology. 2003;**24**:800-806

[49] De Beer L, Stokroos R, Kingma H. Intratympanic gentamicin therapy for intractable Meniere's disease. Acta Oto-Laryngologica. 2007;**127**:605-612

[50] Casani AP, Piaggi P, Cerchiai N, Seccia V, Franceschini SS, Dallan I. Intratympanic treatment of intractable

unilateral Meniere disease: Gentamicin or dexamethasone? A randomized controlled trial. Otolaryngolog—Head and Neck Surgery. 2012;**146**:430-437

[51] Vlastarakos PV, Iacovou E, Nikolopoulos TP. Is gentamycin delivery via sustained-release vehicles a safe and effective treatment for refractory Meniere's disease? A critical analysis of published interventional studies. European Archives of Oto-Rhino-Laryngology. 2017;**274**:1309-1315

[52] Nevoux J, Barbara M, Dornhoffer J, Gibson W, Kitahara T, Darrouzet V. International consensus (ICON) on treatment of Meniere's disease. European Annals of Otorhinolaryngology, Head and Neck Diseases. 2018;**135**:S29-S32

[53] Bauer PW, MacDonald CB, Cox LC. Intratympanic gentamicin therapy for vertigo in nonserviceable ears. American Journal of Otolaryngology. 2001;**22**:111-115

[54] Sajjadi H, Paparella MM. Meniere's disease. Lancet. 2008;**372**:406-414

[55] Marzo SJ, Leonetti JP. Intratympanic gentamicin therapy for persistent vertigo after endolymphatic sac surgery. Otolaryngology—Head and Neck Surgery. 2002;**126**:31-33

[56] Prezant TR, Agapian JV, Bohlman MC, Bu X, Oztas S, Qiu WQ, et al. Mitochondrial ribosomal RNA mutation associated with both antibiotic-induced and non-syndromic deafness. Nature Genetics. 1993;**4**:289-294

[57] Liu YC, Chi FH, Yang TH, Liu TC. Assessment of complications due to intratympanic injections. World Journal of Otorhinolaryngology—Head and Neck Surgery. 2016;**2**:13-16

Section 5

Surgical Treatment

Chapter 6

Surgical Procedures for Ménière's Disease

Ricardo Ferreira Bento and Paula Tardim Lopes

Abstract

The aim of this chapter is to present a literature review on some of the main articles describing different interventions for the treatment in patients with progressive intractable Ménière disease symptoms. Even though each paper presents good results in defending its techniques, there have been few well-designed clinical studies, that is, studies involving control groups or long-term observation, in the efficacy of surgery with respect to vertigo control and hearing preservation. Focusing on presenting the different techniques established in the literature, we discuss the main indications and results obtained regarding the control of vertigo and the audiological outcomes after the procedure. Physicians should offer additional treatment strategies for Meniere's disease patients with a long history of limiting symptoms or associated hearing loss. The surgical options for such patients should be considered carefully because surgery can damage the ipsilateral ear and the hearing function of the contralateral ear is often suboptimal. Its importance is that alternatives for treatment can only be offered to a patient when doctor knows them.

Keywords: Ménière's disease, hearing loss, vertigo, endolymphatic sac, vestibular rehabilitation

1. Introduction

Ménière's disease is a clinical diagnosis based on the 1995 classification by the American Academy of Otolaryngology-Head and Neck Surgery (AAO-HNS) Committee on Hearing and Equilibrium [1]. The definitive diagnosis of Ménière's disease can be made with specific tests such as audiometry and electrocochleography in the exacerbated states of the disease. Recently, a study by Bernaerts [2] showed diagnostic evidences with the use of magnetic resonance imaging (MRI) scans, which showed an enlargement of the perilymphatic spaces in Ménière's disease.

The endolymphatic sac physiologically maintains the hydrostatic pressure and endolymph homeostasis in the inner ear, and its dysfunction may contribute to the pathophysiology of Ménière's disease. The classic tetrad of symptoms in endolymphatic hydrops includes recurrent attacks of vertigo lasting for hours, fluctuating hearing loss, auricular fullness, and tinnitus. Ménière's disease is idiopathic, as its aetiology remains unknown. Over the years, different surgical procedures for intractable vertigo secondary to Ménière's disease have been carried out, and although many authors consider these procedures effective, some argue that they only have a placebo effect. Usually, surgical procedures are indicated in about 20% of the patients when the possibilities of treatment with drugs for vestibular rehabilitation have already been exhausted [3–6].

IntechOpen

The surgical technique for the treatment of vertigo depends on the diagnostic hypothesis, clinical condition, age, and hearing level of the patient.

2. Conservative procedures for Ménière's disease

This chapter describes the different surgical procedures performed for Ménière's disease. They can be divided into two types: non-destructive surgery, aimed at altering the disease expression and at reducing the frequency and intensity of vestibular drop attacks; and destructive surgery, aimed at controlling vertigo by stopping the vestibular function.

The most common procedures are the endolymphatic sac decompression with or without the endolymphatic duct opening and shunt in the endolymphatic sac, endolymphatic duct blockage, and intratympanic corticosteroid injection.

2.1 Endolymphatic sac decompression and shunt in the endolymphatic sac

Decompression of the endolymphatic sac involves reducing pressure in this space. It is considered a conservative procedure because of the low rate of hearing loss and the high success rate (around 80% or more) of vertigo control [7, 8].

The first surgical procedure for the treatment of Ménière's disease was described in 1927 by Portmann [9, 10], who first opened the endolymphatic sac to decrease the endolymphatic pressure. In 1938, Hallpike and Cairns [11] showed the pathological findings of endolymphatic hydrops in post-mortem temporal bones of patients who were also diagnosed with Ménière's disease. These bones showed signs of ischemia in the sensory terminal endings at the lateral walls of the membranous labyrinth, which could have been caused by the presence of hydrops.

In 1962, William House [12] showed that draining endolymphatic hydrops using a subarachnoid shunt had good outcomes. In 1967, Kimura [13] obliterated the endolymph duct and attenuated the endolymphatic hydrops in guinea pigs, following which surgeons innovated new techniques of mastoid shunts. In 1976, Paparella [14] described a technique that emphasised the need to make a wide incision in the dura mater of the posterior fossa to completely decompress the endolymphatic sac and duct, increasing its drainage through a valve created in this duct with the placement of a T-tube.

Paparella described that this surgical technique was a modification of the surgical technique of the endolymphatic sac described by Portmann and showed a 94% control rate for vertigo [15].

In a 2014 meta-analysis conducted by Sood et al. [16], the various endolymphatic surgical techniques were analysed, along with their efficacy in vertigo control and hearing maintenance. The study demonstrated that the decompression procedures of the endolymphatic sac both alone and associated with shunt placement in the mastoid were effective, without any statistical difference in the 75% control of vertigo symptoms in a short period of 12–24 months.

Bento et al. [17] conducted a retrospective study of endolymphatic sac decompression using the retrolabyrinthine approach in 95 patients with Ménière's disease who did not undergo long-term clinical treatment. In the group with unilateral disease, vertigo was controlled in 94.3%, cochlear function significantly improved in 14%, and hearing was preserved or improved in 88% of patients. In the group with bilateral disease, vertigo was controlled in 85.7%, cochlear function improved in 28%, and auditory function was preserved in 71% of patients. Considerable improvement in hearing was an improvement of more than 20 dB in the bone conduction threshold or improvement by more than 20% in the discrimination score (**Figures 1** and 2).

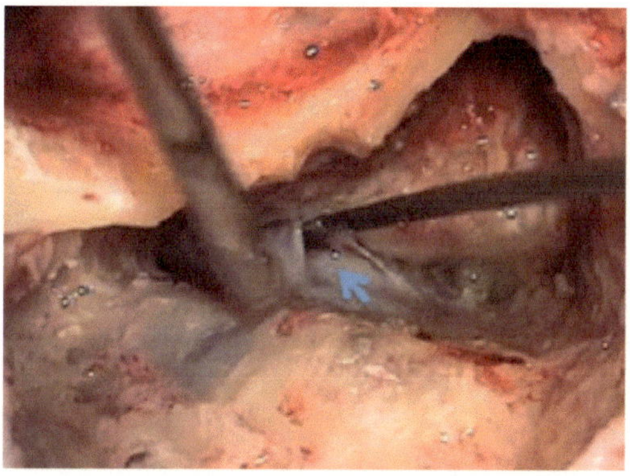

Figure 1.
The sac is opened (arrowhead).

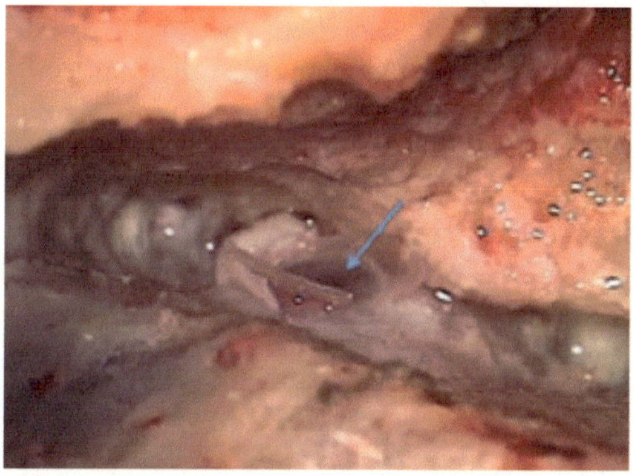

Figure 2.
A silastic sheet (arrow) is placed to keep the sac opened.

The surgical method of endolymphatic sac decompression and drainage of the endolymphatic duct, as previously described by Paparella et al. [18–20], involves a broad exposure of the mastoid cortex, wall-up mastoidectomy, and extensive removal of the pre-sigmoidal and retrolabyrinthine cells.

A very thin skeletal bone should cover the sigmoid sinus, and a small bone island should be left over it to avoid damage from pressure and bleeding. With the Trautmann's triangle fully exposed, the overlying bone is removed with a curette or microdissector, and the sac is then identified as a dense white thickening in the dura mater pointing toward the lower portion of the posterior semicircular canal. Mostly, the sac is clearly differentiated from the adjacent dura mater by its greater thickness in the region and lack of blood vessels. After identifying the endolymphatic sac, a small aperture is created in it with a paracentesis blade or a scalpel, often below the bone border, by retracting the dura mater with a suction tip to expose the lumen. To keep the opening intact, a T-shaped silastic sheet is cut to about 0.127 mm thickness and positioned in the opening, or a T-tube is used. After the procedure, an absorbable gelatine haemostatic sponge is placed in the mastoid cavity, and the wound is closed.

2.2 Endolymphatic duct block

In this technique, the sac is not incised. The surgeon dissects the bone around the endolymphatic duct to expose it and blocks it with two small titanium clips.

The endolymphatic sac gets isolated, so the production and absorption of endolymph in the inner ear balance. Saliba et al. [21] conducted a randomised controlled, non-blinded study comparing this technique with the endolymphatic sac decompression and showed that 96.5% of the patients in the endolymphatic block group achieved vertigo control compared to 37.5% of the patients in the endolymphatic sac decompression group, with no statistical differences between the groups in pre- and post-operative auditory thresholds.

In summary, endolymphatic duct blockade has potential as a surgical technique that results in good control of vertigo.

2.3 Corticosteroid therapy

In 1986, Brookes [22] showed the presence of high levels of circulating immunocomplexes in up to 54% of patients with Ménière's disease. Later, Alleman et al. [23] extracted the circulating immunocomplexes from patients with Ménière's disease and exposed them to endolymphatic sac tissue from other patients with the disease, showing that in only 10% of cases, there was a reaction between the immune complexes and tissues. Hence, it is suggested that although the levels of circulating immunocomplexes in these patients is high, they can represent an induction (viral, allergic, or traumatic) that is greater than an autoimmune phenomenon. Another pathophysiological analysis of Ménière's disease showed that the immune-mediated responses in the inner ear, endolymphatic sac, and vascular striae could be the main causative factors. In 1997, Shea et al. [24] showed that combined administration of systemic and intratympanic dexamethasone completely suppressed vertigo in 63.4% and significantly improved hearing in 35.4% of patients within 2 years after treatment. Later in 2001, Sennaroglu et al. [25] reported that intratympanic perfusion of dexamethasone completely suppressed vertigo in 42.0% and significantly improved hearing in 16% of patients within 2 years after treatment.

3. Destructive surgeries for Ménière's disease

These labyrinthine surgeries cure the patient of vertigo by destroying the final vestibular organ. The brain compensates for the loss of vestibular function on one side using the contralateral labyrinth, as long as it is functioning properly. Destructive labyrinthine procedures have a high risk of destroying the cochlea and should be avoided in patients with adequate hearing. Vestibulocochlear nerve neurectomy, chemical labyrinthectomy, surgical labyrinthectomy, and sacculotomy are common destructive surgeries.

3.1 Vestibulocochlear nerve neurectomy

The neurectomy of the vestibulocochlear nerve for the treatment of Ménière's disease was described in 1933 by Dandy [26]. It is a surgical technique involving a selective section of the vestibular nerve at its entrance to the brain to reduce vertigo but inevitably causing total hearing loss in the operated ear.

Several authors modified the original technique. In 1989, Silverstein [27] proposed the retrosigmoid approach for neurectomy and observed a substantial improvement in dizziness in 92% with a significant hearing loss in only 4% of patients.

House [28] introduced the middle fossa approach. Regardless of the access, the decompression technique had a success rate of up to 90% in the control of vertigo [29–33]. Colletti et al. [4] conducted a comparative study on 209 patients who underwent neurectomy, comparing a group of 24 patients who received intratympanic gentamicin (ITG), chemical labyrinthectomy neural ablation therapy. To perform a homogenous comparison of results in the present paper, it considered all the 24 ITG patients and the last 24 patients who underwent VN from 2000 to 2002 via the retrosigmoid approach.

Vertigo was controlled in 95.8% of neurectomy patients and in 75% of gentamicin patients. Speech discrimination in the neurectomy group was reduced from 85 to 82% and in the gentamicin group from 87% to 65%.

3.2 Chemical labyrinthectomy: intratympanic application of gentamicin in the middle ear

This technique was first used in 1978 by Beck [34, 35] and aims to perform a chemical ablation of the labyrinth to decrease the frequency and intensity of vertigo episodes but can result in hearing loss, as gentamicin is ototoxic and reduces labyrinthine activity. It can be injected directly into the tympanic cavity using a thin needle or applied daily through a Politzer ventilation tube first placed at the tympanic membrane for penetrating the round and oval windows. A study [36] showed 90% efficacy in the cessation of vertigo among 92 patients.

In the 2000 literature review by Blakley et al. [37], 18 articles were found on the techniques of intratympanic injection of gentamicin in the treatment of Ménière's disease. The articles reported high success rates in vertigo treatment, but the technique, dose, duration, and treatment philosophy varied considerably among them. Hearing loss was typically reported in about 30% of patients, and no technique had any significant medical advantage over the other. Until new controlled studies indicate otherwise, this therapy is an alternative treatment for patients with major comorbidities.

3.3 Surgical labyrinthectomy

This technique can decrease vertigo by the total destruction of the labyrinth but leads to total hearing loss in the operated ear.

Lake first described this procedure in 1904 [38], and in the mid-twentieth century, labyrinthectomy was established as a less-invasive alternative to neurectomy of the vestibular nerve [39, 40]. The surgical technique involves opening the semicircular canals up to the endolymphatic ducts in the opening of the vestibule with the complete destruction of neuroepithelium and Scarpa's ganglion [41, 42]. No technique was observed to be superior in vertigo control among labyrinthectomy, neurectomy, and a combination of both [43, 44].

Labyrinthectomy, in particular, is an alternative [45] (demonstrating approximately 100% success rate in vertigo treatment) for old patients, and in this case, the transmastoid technique presented a lower permanent imbalance rate after the procedure than the transcanal technique. Labyrinthectomy is the treatment of choice for patients over 60 years of age [46]. Surgical labyrinthectomy of the affected labyrinth always ends in total deafness. Therefore, it should be reserved for patients with non-functional hearing and should be one of the last therapeutic options (**Figure 3**).

3.4 Sacculotomy

In 1964, Fick [47, 48] described a procedure in which a fenestra is made in the stapes footplate or round window membrane, and therefore, a permanent shunt for draining of the saccule is created with the destruction of the cochlear function [49].

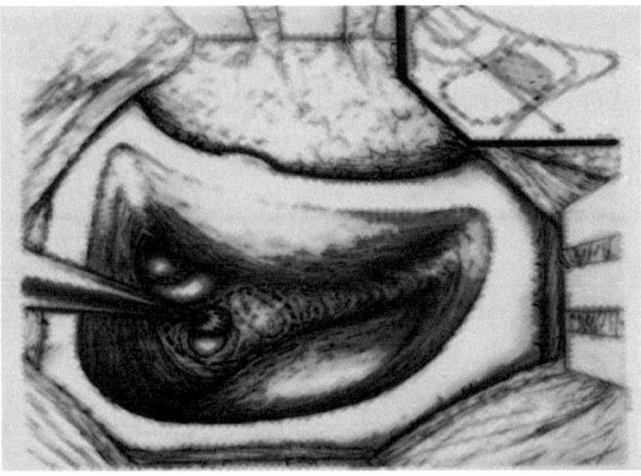

Figure 3.
Schematic drawing of Labyrinthectomy.

Giddings et al. [50] reported hearing loss after cochleo-sacculotomy in 80% of the patients and recurrent vertigo episodes in a mean follow-up of 17 months in 4 of 11 patients so that a destructive intervention had to be carried out again. Kinney et al. [51] and Wielinga et al. [52] recommended cochleo-sacculotomy as a minimally invasive surgical method, especially for old patients, as an alternative to neurectomy because good results were obtained with regard to vertigo control, although with significant hearing loss in almost all patients.

In 2015, in a comparative study [53] between cochlear sacculotomy techniques and endolymphatic sac decompression, the control of vertigo was significantly better in patients after cochleo-sacculotomy but also with significant deterioration of hearing. The cochleo-sacculotomy procedure performed simultaneously with cochlear implant surgery in patients with deafness and persistent vertigo in Ménière's disease is an alternative already proposed by some authors [54–56], and they have reported good results.

4. Conclusion

The surgical procedures described in this chapter demonstrated satisfactory results in the control of incapacitating vertigo in patients diagnosed with endolymphatic hydrops refractory to clinical drug treatment, adequate diet, and vestibular rehabilitation. The choice of method would depend on the quality of residual hearing, contralateral hearing, and on the ability to develop compensatory mechanisms if surgical techniques destroyed vestibular function.

Conflict of interest

The authors have no conflict of interest.

Author details

Ricardo Ferreira Bento and Paula Tardim Lopes*
Department of Otorhinolaryngology and Neurotology, Hospital das Clínicas—University of São Paulo, São Paulo, Brazil

*Address all correspondence to: paula.tardim@hc.fm.usp.br

References

[1] Committee on Hearing and Equilibrium. Committee on hearing and equilibrium guidelines for the diagnosis and evaluation of therapy in Meniere's disease. American Academy of Otolaryngology—Head and Neck Foundation, Inc. Otolaryngology and Head and Neck Surgery. 1995;**113**(3):181-185

[2] Bernaerts A, Vanspauwen R, Blaivie C, et al. The value of four stage vestibular hydrops grading and asymmetric perilymphatic enhancement in the diagnosis of Menière's disease on MRI. Neuroradiology. 2019;**61**(4):421-429. DOI: 10.1007/s00234-019-02155-7

[3] Liston SL, Nissen RL, Paparella MM, Da Costa SS. Surgical treatment of vertigo. In: Paparella MM, Shumrick DA, Gluckman JL, Meyerhoff WL, editors. Otolaryngology. Volume II. Philadelphia: WB Saunders Company; 1991. pp. 1715-1732

[4] Colletti V, Carner M, Colletti L. Auditory results after vestibular nerve section and intratympanic gentamicin for Ménière's disease. Otology & Neurotology. 2007;**28**(2):145-151. DOI: 10.1097/MAO.0b013e31802c7989

[5] Sajjadi H, Paparella MM. Ménière's disease. Lancet. 2008;**372**(9636): 406-414. DOI: 10.1016/S0140-6736(08)61161-7

[6] Yokota Y, Kitahara T, Sakagami M, Ito T, Kimura T, Okayasu T, et al. Surgical results and psychological status in patients with intractable Ménière's disease. Auris, Nasus, Larynx. 2016;**43**(3):287-291. DOI: 10.1016/j.anl.2015.10.007

[7] Brinson GM, Chen DA, Arriaga MA. Endolymphatic mastoid shunt versus endolymphatic sac decompression for Ménière's disease. Otolaryngology and Head and Neck Surgery. 2007;**136**(3):415-421. DOI: 10.1016/j.otohns.2006.08.031

[8] Kitahara T, Horii A, Imai T, Ohta Y, Morihana T, Inohara H, et al. Effects of endolymphatic sac decompression surgery on vertigo and hearing in patients with bilateral Ménière's disease. Otology & Neurotology. 2014;**35**(10):1852-1857. DOI: 10.1097/MAO.0000000000000469

[9] Portmann G. The saccus endolinphaticus and the operation for draining the same for relief of vertigo. The Journal of Laryngology and Otology. 1927;**42**:809-817

[10] Portamann G. Surgical treatment of vertigo by opening of the saccus endolymphaticus. Archives of Otolaryngology. 1969;**89**(6):809-815

[11] Hallpike CS, Cairns H. Observation on pathology of Ménière's syndrome. The Journal of Laryngology and Otology. 1938;**53**:624-654

[12] House WF. Subarachnoid shunt for drainage of endolymphatic hydrops. A preliminary report. Laryngoscope. 1962;**72**:713-729. DOI: 10.1288/00005537-196206000-00003

[13] Kimura RS. Experimental blockage of the endolymphatic duct and sac and its effects on the inner ear of the guinea pig. A study on endolymphatic hydrops. The Annals of Otology, Rhinology, and Laryngology. 1967;**76**(3):664-687. DOI: 10.1177/000348946707600311

[14] Paparella MM, Hanson DG. Endolymphatic sac drainage for intractable vertigo (method and experiences). The Laryngoscope. 1976;**86**(5):697-703. DOI: 10.1288/00005537-197605000-00010

[15] Paparella MM, Goycoolea M. Panel of Menière's disease. Endolymphatic sac enhancement surgery for Menière's disease: An extension of conservative therapy. The Annals of Otology, Rhinology, and Laryngology. 1981;**90**(6 Pt 1):610-615. DOI: 10.1177/000348948109000620

[16] Sood AJ, Lambert PR, Nguyen SA, Meyer TA. Endolymphatic sac surgery for Ménière's disease: A systematic review and meta-analysis. Otology & Neurotology. 2014;**35**(6):1033-1045. DOI: 10.1097/MAO.0000000000000324

[17] Bento RF, Cisneros JC, De Oliveira Fonseca AC. Endolymphatic sac drainage for the treatment of Ménière's disease. The Journal of Laryngology and Otology. 2016;**131**(2):144-149. DOI: 10.1017/S0022215116009713

[18] Paparella MM, Goycoolea M. Panel of Ménière's disease. Endolymphatic sac enhancement surgery for Ménière's disease: An extension of conservative therapy. The Annals of Otology, Rhinology, and Laryngology. 1981;**90**(6 Pt 1):610-615. DOI: 10.1177/000348948109000620

[19] Paparella MM, Sajjadi H. Endolymphatic sac enhancement. Otolaryngologic Clinics of North America. 1994;**27**(2):381-402

[20] Paparella MM. Revision of endolymphatic sac surgery for recurrent Ménière's disease. Otolaryngologic Clinics of North America. 2002;**35**(3):607-619

[21] Saliba I, Gabra N, Alzahrani M, Berbiche D. Endolymphatic duct blockage: A randomized controlled trial of a novel surgical technique for Ménière's disease treatment. Otolaryngology and Head and Neck Surgery. 2015;**152**(1):122-129. DOI: 10.1177/0194599814555840

[22] Brookes GB. Circulating immune complexes in Meniere's disease. Archives of Otolaryngology—Head & Neck Surgery. 1986;**112**(5):536-540

[23] Alleman AM, Dornhoffer JL, Arenberg IK, Walker PD. Demonstration of autoantibodies to the endolymphatic sac in Meniere's disease. The Laryngoscope. 1997;**107**(2):211-215

[24] Shea JJ Jr. The role of dexamethasone or streptomycin perfusion in the treatment of Meniere's disease. Otolaryngologic Clinics of North America. 1997;**30**(6):1051-1059

[25] Sennaroglu L, Sennaroglu G, Gursel B, Dini FM. Intratympanic dexamethasone, intratympanic gentamicin, and endolymphatic sac surgery for intractable vertigo in Meniere's disease. Otolaryngology and Head and Neck Surgery. 2001;**125**(5):537-543. DOI: 10.1067/mhn.2001.119485

[26] Dandy WE. Treatment of Meniere's disease by section of only the vestibular portion of the acoustic nerve. Bulletin of the Johns Hopkins Hospital. 1933;**53**:52-55

[27] Silverstein H, Jackson LE. Vestibular nerve section. Otolaryngologic Clinics of North America. 2002;**35**(3):655-673

[28] House WF. Surgical exposure of the internal auditory canal and its contents through the middle cranial fossa. The Laryngoscope. 1961;**71**:1363-1385. DOI: 10.1288/00005537-196111000-00004

[29] Reid CB, Eisenberg R, Halmagyi GM, Fagan PA. The outcome of vestibular nerve section for intractable vertigo: The patient's point of view. The Laryngoscope. 1996;**106** (12 Pt 1):1553-1556

[30] Pappas DG Jr, Pappas DG Sr. Vestibular nerve section: Long-term

follow-up. The Laryngoscope. 1997;**107**(9):1203-1209

[31] De Diego JI, Prim MP, Melcon E, de Sarriá MJ, Gavilán J. Result of middle fossa vestibular neurectomy in Meniere's disease. Acta Otorrinolaringológica Española. 2001;**52**(4):283-286

[32] Nakahara H, Takemori S, Seki Y, Umezu H. Hearing changes and questionnaire responses in patients with paramedian suboccipital vestibular neurectomy. Acta Oto-Laryngologica. Supplementum. 2001;**545**:108-112

[33] Schlegel M, Vibert D, Ott SR, Häusler R, Caversaccio MD. Functional results and quality of life after retrosigmoid vestibular neurectomy in patients with Ménière's disease. Otology & Neurotology. 2012;**33**(8):1380-1385

[34] Beck C, Schmidt CL. 10 years of experience with intratympanally applied streptomycin (gentamycin) in the therapy of morbus Meniere. Archives of Oto-Rhino-Laryngology. 1978;**221**(2):149-152

[35] Beck C. Intratympanic application of gentamicin for treatment of Meniere's disease. The Keio Journal of Medicine. 1986;**35**(1):36-41

[36] Lange G. Gentamicin and other ototoxic antibiotics for the transtympanic treatment for Meniere's disease. Archives of Oto-Rhino-Laryngology. 1989;**246**(5):269-270

[37] Blakley BW. Update on intratympanic gentamicin for Meniere's disease. The Laryngoscope. 2000;**110** (2 Pt 1):236-240

[38] Lake R. Removal of the semicircular canals in a case of unilateral aural vertigo. Lancet. 1904;**1**:1567-1568

[39] Cawthorne TE, Hallpike CS. Some recent work on the investigation and treatment of "Ménière's" disease. Proceedings of the Royal Society of Medicine. 1943;**36**(10):533-550

[40] Day KM. Surgical treatment of hydrops of the labyrinth; surgical destruction of the labyrinth for Ménière's disease. The Laryngoscope. 1952;**62**(6):547-555

[41] Jones R, Silverstein H, Smouha E. Long-term results of transmeatal cochleovestibular neurectomy: An analysis of 100 cases. Otolaryngology and Head and Neck Surgery. 1989;**100**(1):22-29

[42] Langman AW, Lindeman RC. Surgery for vertigo in the nonserviceable hearing ear: Transmastoid labyrinthectomy or translabyrinthine vestibular nerve section. The Laryngoscope. 1993;**103**(12):1321-1325

[43] Gacek RR, Gacek MR. Comparison of labyrinthectomy and vestibular neurectomy in the control of vertigo. The Laryngoscope. 1996;**106**(2 Pt 1): 225-230

[44] Eisenman DJ, Speers R, Telian SA. Labyrinthectomy versus vestibular neurectomy: Long-term physiologic and clinical outcomes. Otology & Neurotology. 2001;**22**(4):539-548

[45] Schwaber MK, Pensak ML, Reiber ME. Transmastoid labyrinthectomy in older patients. The Laryngoscope. 1995;**105**(11):1152-1154

[46] Langman AW, Lindeman RC. Surgical labyrinthectomy in the older patient. Otolaryngology and Head and Neck Surgery. 1998;**118**:739-742

[47] Fick IA. Decompression of the labyrinth: A new surgical procedure for Meniere's disease. Archives of Otolaryngology. 1964;**79**:447-458

[48] van Fick IA. Symposium: Management of Ménière's disease. VI. Sacculotomy for hydrops. The Laryngoscope. 1965;**75**(10):1539-1546

[49] Schuknecht HF. Cochleosacculotomy for Meniere's disease: Theory, technique and results. The Laryngoscope. 1982;**92**(8 Pt 1):853-858

[50] Giddings NA, Shelton C, O'Leary MJ, Brackmann DE. Cochleosacculotomy revisited: Long-term results poorer than expected. Archives of Otolaryngology—Head & Neck Surgery. 1991;**117**(10):1150-1152

[51] Kinney WC, Nalepa N, Hughes GB, Kinney SE. Cochleosacculotomy for the treatment of Menière's disease in the elderly patient. The Laryngoscope. 1995;**105**(9 Pt 1):934-937

[52] Wielinga EW, Smyth GD. Long-term results of sacculotomy in older patients. The Annals of Otology, Rhinology, and Laryngology. 1989;**98**(10):803-806

[53] Soheilipour S, Abtahi SH, Soltani M, Khodadadi HA. Comparison the results of two different vestibular system surgery in patients with persistent Meniere's disease. Advanced Biomedical Research. 2015;**4**:198. DOI: 10.4103/2277-9175.166134

[54] Mukherjee P, Eykamp K, Brown D, Curthoys I, Flanagan S, Biggs N, et al. Cochlear implantation in Ménière's disease with and without labyrinthectomy. Otology & Neurotology. 2017;**38**(2):192-198. DOI: 10.1097/MAO.0000000000001278

[55] Prenzler NK, Bültmann E, Giourgas A, Steffens M, Salcher RB, Stolle S, et al. Cochlear implantation in patients with definite Meniere's disease. European Archives of Oto-Rhino-Laryngology. 2017;**274**(2):751-756. DOI: 10.1007/s00405-016-4356-z

[56] Heywood RL, Atlas MD. Simultaneous cochlear implantation and labyrinthectomy for advanced Ménière's disease. The Journal of Laryngology and Otology. 2016;**130**(2):204-206. DOI: 10.1017/S0022215115003345

Section 6

Future of Surgical Treatment

Chapter 7

Meniere's Disease: Surgical Treatment

Yetkin Zeki Yilmaz, Begum Bahar Yilmaz and Mehmet Yilmaz

Abstract

When Meniere's disease's vertigo attacks are too frequent and medical treatment options fail, surgical treatment options should be considered. Meniere's disease is progressive, and there is not a known cure, and all treatment options are symptomatic. Also the possibility of bilateral involvement is another well-known characteristic of this condition as well as its effect on hearing. Some of the patients have progressive hearing loss with vertigo attacks. In order to decide a surgical procedure for these patients, clinicians must be aware of the natural course of Meniere's disease. In order to their effects on vestibular system, there are two types of surgical procedures. Nondestructive surgeries aim to alter the course of disease, and destructive surgeries aim to control symptoms while eliminating all vestibular functions of the effected ear.

Keywords: Meniere's disease, labyrinthectomy, vestibular neurectomy, endolymphatic sac surgery, neuro-otology

1. Introduction

When Meniere's disease's vertigo attacks are too frequent and medical treatment options fail, surgical treatment options should be considered. Meniere's disease is progressive; there is not a known cure and all treatment options are symptomatic. Also the possibility of bilateral involvement is another well-known characteristic of this condition as well as its effect on hearing. Some of the patients have progressive hearing loss with vertigo attacks. In order to decide a surgical procedure for these patients, clinicians must be aware of the natural course of Meniere's disease.

Some authors recommend to wait 6–12 months in order to recommend surgery for intractable Meniere's disease. However, there are different definitions of "intractability." When medical treatment fails and patient keep experiencing severe and frequent vertigo attacks, surgery option could be evaluated. If the symptoms are resistant to medical and psychological therapy for at least 3–6 months, hearing loss and vertigo attacks are frequent, and the condition could be accepted as intractable [1]. Ten to twenty percent of Meniere's disease patients are considered to have an intractable disease [2].

There are destructive and nondestructive surgical options; in decision process, patients' general health condition, age, and hearing levels should be considered. Progressive and bilateral nature of the disease always should be considered.

The ideal surgery must restore remaining functions while relieving patients' severe symptoms. International Consensus (ICON) on treatment of Meniere's

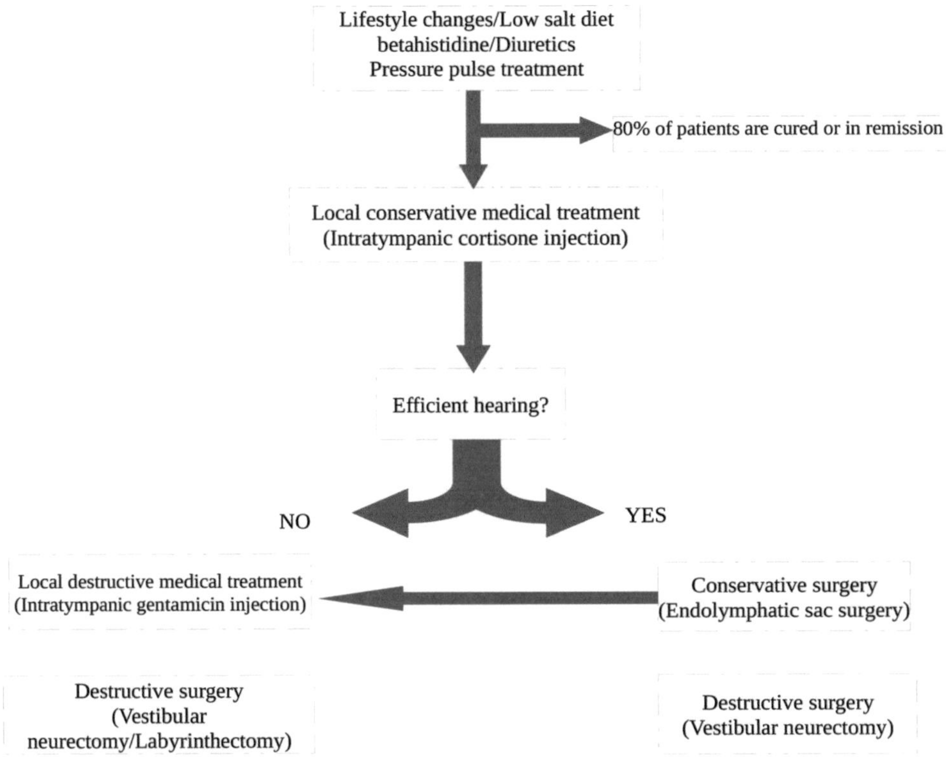

Figure 1.
Treatment algorithm of Meniere's disease, proposed by ICON in 2018.

disease recently proposed a treatment algorithm. When conservatory treatment options were insufficient to control patient's symptoms, it is recommended to evaluate patient's remaining hearing. If the effected ear has efficient hearing, conservative surgical treatment options are recommended, but if remained hearing is not efficient, destructive surgical or medical treatment options are recommended. Conservative surgery is the third step of the treatment, while destructive surgery is the fifth and last option (**Figure 1**) [3].

French Otorhinolaryngology Head and Neck Surgery Society (SFORL)'s guideline of Meniere's disease recommends surgical options after noninvasive treatment options were tried [4]. European position statement on diagnosis and treatment of Meniere's disease has similar opinions about surgery with ICON and SFORL guidelines [5].

Since local destructive medical treatment (intratympanic gentamicin) is another subject of another chapter of this book, the main focus of this chapter will be surgical procedures.

2. Patient selection

A successful treatment requires precise diagnosis. Typical Meniere's disease causes fluctuating hearing loss and episodic vertigo that could last minutes to hours with tinnitus and ear fullness. For every patient who describes one or more of these symptoms, clinician should consider Meniere's disease in differential diagnosis. Even nowadays, diagnosis of Meniere's disease is clinical. Detailed history and complete physical examination should be taken. After routine exam, there are some diagnostic tests that should be ordered like complete audiometric assessment, vestibular test battery, and imaging studies. Differential diagnosis of unilateral vestibular disorders is summarized in **Table 1**.

MR imaging studies should be ordered in all unilateral cases of Meniere's disease. It is helpful to exclude retrocochlear pathologies, endolymphatic sac tumors, vestibular schwannomas, or any other conditions that could mimic the symptoms of Meniere's disease. Also Nakashima et al. managed to visualize endolymphatic hydrops in Meniere's disease after administrating the contrast substance gadolinium intratympanically [6]. Miyagawa et al. visualized the endolymphatic hydrops with intravenous administered gadolinium MRI [7]. Naganawa and Nakashima evaluated the imaging for Meniere's disease and its correlation with vestibular tests of Meniere's disease patients. They reported that endolymphatic hydrops could be observed with MRI, and also all patients with Meniere's disease had endolymphatic hydrops in imaging studies, but not all patients who had endolymphatic hydrops were diagnosed with Meniere's disease [8]. If patient is unable to go under MRI, auditory brainstem response audiometry could be helpful to evaluate retrocochlear pathologies [9]. Nevertheless imaging studies are important part of differential diagnosis; also if surgery is going to be performed, computed tomography should be ordered for surgery plan.

Serial audiograms are helpful to document fluctuating hearing loss. Most specific pattern is sensorineural hearing loss of low frequency and its reversibility. Most authors reported sensorineural hearing loss at low frequencies with better hearing at 2000 Hz, called peak pattern [10, 11].

Unilateral vestibular hypofunction is most common finding of unilateral Meniere's disease, although it is reported that half of the Meniere's disease patients have completely normal responses in bithermal caloric tests [12]. Video head impulse test (VHIT) is a significant parameter to evaluate peripheral vestibular system since it evaluates semicircular canals individually. In order to evaluate utricule and saccule functions, vestibular evoked myogenic potentials (VEMPs) are very useful [13].

Electrocochleography is considered to be the most valuable test to diagnose Meniere's disease. Summation and action potentials that arise from cochlea are

Autosomal dominant sensorineural hearing loss type 9 (DFNA9) caused by COCH gene
Autosomal dominant sensorineural hearing loss type 6/14 (DFNA6/14) caused by WSF1 gene
Autoimmune inner ear disease
Cerebrovascular disease (stroke or transient ischemic attack in the vertebrobasilar system, bleeding)
Cogan's syndrome
Endolymphatic sac tumor
Cerebellopontine tumors (such as meningioma)
Neuroborreliosis
Otosyphilis
Susac syndrome
Third window syndromes (perilymph fistula, canal dehiscence, enlarged vestibular aqueduct)
Vestibular migraine
Vestibular schwannoma
Vogt-Koyanagi-Harada syndrome

Table 1.
Differential diagnosis of unilateral vestibular disorders.

Peripheral labyrinth dysfunction	• Unilateral caloric weakness • Spontaneous or positional nystagmus (although oculomotor findings are normal) • Nystagmus could be provoked with specific maneuvers (Dix-Hallpike, Roll, etc.) • Asymmetric or abnormal rotational chair phase • Reduced gain on rotational chair phase (bilateral weakness)
Central nervous system pathology	• Vertical or perverted nystagmus • Abnormal oculomotor test results • Nystagmus would not be suppressed with visual fixation
Uncompensation	• Persistent nystagmus (positional or spontaneous) • Post head-shaking nystagmus • Asymmetric rotational chair phase • Abnormal dynamic posturography
Compensation	• Resolution of nystagmus • Resolution of asymmetric rotational chair phase • Improvement of performance on dynamic posturography

Table 2.
Clinical interpretations of vestibular tests.

evaluated. Summation potential/action potential ratio increases in order of endolymphatic hydrops [14]. It is not diagnostic for Meniere's disease; the ratio is found to be elevated at 62% of Meniere's disease patients as well as 21% of control subjects [15].

Sixty to eighty-seven percent of patients with Meniere's disease reported to be able to continue their normal life style with medical treatment [16, 17]. If medical treatment tried for 3–6 months and attacks of patient was not able to be controlled with medical treatment, surgical options must be considered [18, 19]. Character of the surgery is decided upon patient's remaining hearing. If hearing levels are 50 dB or higher or speech discrimination scores are 80% or higher, conservative surgeries should be offered, but if hearing is not functional, destructive options must be considered [20].

The interpretation of vestibular test results was summarized in **Table 2**.

3. Surgical procedures

In order to their effects on vestibular system, there are two types of surgical procedures. Nondestructive surgeries aim to alter the course of disease, and destructive surgeries aim to control symptoms while eliminating all vestibular functions of the effected ear.

Nondestructive procedures are endolymphatic sac decompression or shunt in order to increase endolymph drainage, ventilation tube insertion in order to equalize increased pressure of inner and middle ear, and lateral semicircular canal plugging to block the movement of endolymph into the effected canal [21].

Destructive procedures aim to abolish the end vestibular organs. Most of these procedures have high risk to harm the cochlea. Selective vestibular neurectomy aims to cut all the inputs coming from vestibular organs, cochleovestibular nerve section aims to stop all vestibular and audiologic input from the effected ear, labyrinthectomy aims to destruct the labyrinth which also leads to total hearing loss of the operated side, and chemical ablation aims to abolish vestibular inputs, which also has a risk to cause hearing loss and will be evaluated in another chapter [22].

3.1 Nondestructive procedures

3.1.1 Cochleosacculotomy

Cochleosacculotomy is also called "cochlear endolymphatic shunt procedure." This procedure's aim is to equalize the pressure between the perilymph and endolymph by creating a permanent shunt [23].

3.1.1.1 Definition of the procedure

Tympanomeatal flap is elevated and a round window niche is visualized. Angled pick is inserted through the round window membrane and directed to the oval window, and then osseous spiral lamina of cochlea is fractured.

3.1.1.2 Indications and complications

This procedure is rather easy when compared to other surgeries. It does not have risk of cerebrospinal fluid leakage. However, sensorineural hearing loss is expected to be 25% on high-frequency sensorineural hearing loss and 10% of profound hearing loss are reported [24]. Success rates are up to 70% with long-term vertigo relief [25]. It should be considered as an alternative of labyrinthectomy in elder patient who already had severe hearing loss [26].

3.1.2 Endolymphatic sac surgery

The exact pathophysiology of Meniere's disease is still unclear, but one of the most accepted theories is endolymphatic hydrops. Temporal bone studies of Meniere's disease patients reported endolymphatic hydrops [27, 28]. The AAO-HNS guideline of Meniere's disease defines "certain" Meniere's disease when endolymphatic hydrops are demonstrated histopathologically in the postmortem temporal bone specimen of the patient [29].

Endolymph is produced in stria vascularis and dark vestibular cells. It flows through the duct to the sac, and with active transport mechanisms, it is absorbed [30]. Animal study designed by Kimura et al. achieved to cause cochlear hydrops by ductus reuniens obliteration [31].

Paparella suggested that inadequate absorption of endolymph leads to endolymphatic hydrops. He described his theory with "lake-river-pond" comparison while endolymphatic sac is the pond, vestibular aqueduct is the river, and endolymphatic space is the lake. Any obstruction or overproduction leads to hydrops [32]. Perisaccular fibrosis, endolymphatic sac atrophy, loss of epithelial integrity of endolymphatic sac, vestibular aqueduct hypoplasia, and narrowing of endolymphatic duct lumen were observed in the pathological findings in temporal bone studies [30, 33–35].

Also some anatomic abnormalities were observed during endolymphatic sac procedures and proposed as a cause of hydrops. Some of the patient's lateral semicircular canal are located anteriorly and observed in many of the patients. It was suggested to cause vascular compression of endolymphatic sac that leads to hydrops [36, 37].

The findings of revision endolymphatic sac surgeries are another source that used to gather information about the pathophysiology of the disease. Hypoplastic mastoid air cell system with perisaccular fibrosis, discoloration of silastic tube that is inserted at primer surgery, incomplete decompression of sigmoid sinus and mastoid cavity, granulation formation in mastoid cavity, and perisaccular space were the reported findings [36–38].

Portmann was the first surgeon who suggested endolymphatic sac surgery for Meniere's disease nearly 90 years ago and reported improvement of hearing and vestibular functions of patients [39]. In the 1960s, House suggested endolymphatic subarachnoid shunt procedure [40]. Endolymphatic sac enhancement to mastoid cavity was proposed by Paparella et al. in 1980 [41].

3.1.2.1 Definition of the procedure

First cortical mastoidectomy is performed and carried on until the mastoid antrum is visualized. Then the bony labyrinth should be identified. Horizontal and superior semicircular canals are important landmarks of this procedure. Imaginary line that parallel to the horizontal semicircular canal toward to the dome of the superior semicircular canal is called "Donaldson line" is drawn. Endolymphatic sac is always located inferior of this line.

Boundaries of the endolymphatic sac are Donaldson line in superior, sigmoid sinus in posterior, jugular bulb in anteroinferior, and mastoid segment of facial nerve in lateral. These structures are in danger during this procedure. Sigmoid sinus should be skeletonized widely and facial nerve should be followed toward the digastric ridge and stylomastoid foramen in order to avoid to harm these structures. Posterior fossa dura behind the sigmoid sinus as well as the sigmoid sinus is decompressed with a large diamond drill.

Sigmoid sinus is retracted and bony dural plate and presigmoid posterior fossa dura is dissected. The sigmoid sinus and dura are retracted, and the bony dural plate that is located inferior of the Donaldson line is removed to the jugular bulb. In order to see the endolymphatic duct's entry in to bone medial to posterior semicircular canal, dissection should be carried anteromedially into retrofacial air cells. When the endolymphatic sac is identified, it is up to the surgeon to terminate the procedure or open the lumen and place a shunt. Shunt could be placed into mastoid cavity of subarachnoid space.

This procedure has many variations, sac decompression with or without decompression of posterior fossa dura or sigmoid sinus and sac drainage or shunt placement to sac [42, 43].

The role of endolymphatic sac in development of Meniere's disease is still unknown. Inadequate absorption of endolymph by the endolymphatic sac hypothetically causes hydrops which leads to Meniere's disease. The aim of decompression of the sac is to relieve the pressure that inhibits the absorptive capacity of the sac. However, when the temporal bones of patients who underwent endolymphatic sac decompression surgery were studied histopathologically by Chung et al., they observed a diffuse hydrops of the cochlea, saccule, utricule, and ampulla and reported that the decompression is the opposite of the aim of the surgery, not efficient to relieve the hydrops [44]. Linthicum and Santos reported that complete endolymphatic sac removal does not lead to hydrops in the endolymphatic duct or cochlea [45]. According to these findings, Saliba et al. recently described a novel method, endolymphatic sac blockage. They described their procedure in their recently published paper in 2015. Procedure is similar with endolymphatic sac decompression surgery; after the endolymphatic sac identification, they block the endolymphatic duct with two titanium clips. The results were found significantly better than the endolymphatic sac decompression [46].

3.1.2.2 Indications and complications

If medical treatment options failed and hearing function of the patient is sufficient and patient is relatively young, endolymphatic sac surgery should be recommended [3]. Its effect on hearing is minimal and recommended especially in bilateral Meniere's disease [4]. Possible complications are facial paralysis, CSF leak, and hearing loss. Also in order to reach to the endolymphatic sac, the drilling is close to the posterior semicircular canal, so surgery could stimulate the otolith displacement that leads to benign paroxysmal vertigo.

3.1.2.3 Results

The results of this procedure are mostly from retrospective or observational studies. It is usually reported as an efficient and relatively safe procedure. However most of the studies lack randomization or placebo control.

The rate of complete control of vertigo after endolymphatic sac surgery is reported to be 30–72% in literature [47–52].

Thomsen, Bretlau et al. designed a randomized controlled trial to observe the efficacy of endolymphatic sac surgery. They performed endolymphatic sac surgery and cortical mastoidectomy as placebo procedure on intractable Meniere's disease patients. The results were like a milestone in otology society. Endolymphatic sac surgery results were the same with placebo surgery [2]. This paper decreased the popularity of the procedure. Twenty years later, Welling and Nagaraja re-examined their results. They found that patients who underwent placebo procedure had a complete cortical mastoidectomy when the Trautmann triangle was decompressed. Thomsen and colleagues had completed the most important step of successful decompression surgery, a complete mastoidectomy, in placebo group. After these findings, data was re-analyzed, and it was reported that endolymphatic sac surgery results on vertigo control and hearing preservation in short term were significantly better than the placebo procedure [53].

Ostrowski et al. reported that 72% of their patients were significantly improved in long term [43]. Very large group of patients, 3000, had over 90% complete or substantial control of vertigo after 3 years of endolymphatic sac decompression [54].

Kitahara et al. reported that vertigo attacks of patients who received endolymphatic sac surgery, with intraendolymphatic sac steroid injection, had significantly declined, compared to the patients who refused surgery, after 12 years of observation [55].

Cochrane review on surgery for Meniere's disease in 2013 analyzed the literature. Only two studies were suitable for inclusion. Neither of these studies' results were significantly effective on Meniere's disease symptom control, and they reported that the recent data was insufficient in order to demonstrate the benefits of endolymphatic sac surgery [56].

Sood et al. published a meta-analysis on endolymphatic sac surgery procedures. They compared the results of decompression, mastoid shunt with silastic tube and without silastic tube, in short- and long term. Decompression or shunt procedures were found to have similar vertigo control rates in short term, and the same results were observed in long term. Also no significant difference was reported between shunting procedures with or without silastic tube usage. Rates of vertigo control or hearing preservation were found similar between these procedures in short and long term. However hearing preservation results were significantly better in shunting without silastic in short- and long term.

Shunting and decompression have similar effects, but the usage of silastic tube for shunting procedure is not advised [57].

Silverstein compared the results of 83 patients who received endolymphatic sac surgery, vestibular neurectomy, and labyrinthectomy to 50 patients who were surgical candidates but refused the intervention. About 70% of patients who refused the surgery found to be freed of their vertigo attacks in 8.3 years [48].

Saliba et al. described a new approach by blocking the endolymphatic duct. They randomly distributed patients in to two groups, and endolymphatic sac decompression and endolymphatic blockage were performed. They compared the results of endolymphatic sac decompression and endolymphatic duct blockage. After 24 months of follow-up endolymphatic duct blockage group's vertigo spells were significantly improved. Also tinnitus and aural fullness were improved significantly [46].

The results of these procedures may vary between authors, but due to its relatively conservative nature and low complication rates, endolymphatic sac procedures were advised as first line of surgical treatment of intractable Meniere's disease.

3.2 Destructive surgical procedures

When the medical or nondestructive surgical procedures are not able to control the vertigo or after these interventions vertigo is recurrent destruction of the effected side must be considered. Destruction of the labyrinth is the gold standard procedure in order to relieve the patient whose vertigo is caused by an inner ear problem. Remaining hearing is lost completely after labyrinthectomy. If hearing must be preserved, selective vestibular neurectomy should be considered. Both of these procedures' aim is to block any input that come from the defective side.

While blocking the input from the periphery, it is important to prepare the central for better compensation. Before offering any surgical intervention to the vestibular system, adequate vestibular rehabilitation should be tried. After labyrinthectomy or neurectomy, complete unilateral vestibular loss is created. It has been reported that early vestibular rehabilitation after vestibular neurectomy for acoustic neuroma showed improved results to adapt [58–60]. The pathology is different with Meniere's disease, but the result of the ablative procedures is similar. It is an accepted practice to improve the daily functions of the patients. The program should be customized for each patient. Somatosensory sensation is found to be adapted earlier, and within 3 weeks, the sensation of disequilibrium resolves, but gaining of postural stability may take months [61].

Patients' mental state is another important factor that affects the success of the treatment. Patients who had no mental stress found to have better results, compared to stressed ones. Also surgical interventions are found to have better results that nonsurgical treatment in psychologically affected group. The patients' state of mind is an important factor to be considered, and psychological support should be advised to all Meniere's disease effected patients [62]. Patients who have psychological stress like depression, vestibular rehabilitation might be helpful in diagnostic process. This program could help compensation of the remaining vestibular disorder as well as coping with its effects on their psychology. If rehabilitation fails after 4–6 weeks of trial, an unstable vestibular lesion should be added in the differential diagnosis list [63].

Ablative procedures are irreversible, and surgeon must carefully evaluate the patient. Documentation of the symptoms is important to guide the patient to the most appropriate treatment option. Further vestibular investigation should be performed with every patient. These tests provide very useful information on the location of the pathology, labyrinth dysfunction, and compensation statuses.

The observation of spontaneous, positional nystagmus with electronystagmography or videonystagmography means failure of central compensation. In case of an uncompensated peripheral vestibular lesion, vestibuloocular reflex results are persistently asymmetric after several tests. Resolation of this asymmetry is a clue of compensation. Dynamic posturography could provide additional information about all systems that contribute to balance, like vision and somatosensory sense. When the test results are indicating a peripheral vestibular pathology, the offended side must be identified.

Unilateral caloric weakness, under normal oculomotor condition if spontaneous or positional nystagmus is observed, positional nystagmus that provoked with Dix-Hallpike maneuver, asymmetric findings on vestibular tests are indicate to a peripheral labyrinth dysfunction. If nystagmus is persistent, asymmetric results are present rotational chair test or dynamic posturography results indicate an abnormal sensory organization, patient is in an uncompensated status, however if nystagmus, asymmetrics results resolve or posturography performance is improving, compensation status of the patient is improving with the advised treatment method.

Asymmetric sensorineural hearing loss is the best indicator to identify the affected side [64]. The other helpful but less reliable findings are tinnitus, aural fullness, the side that trigger the nystagmus, or asymmetric results from vestibular test batteries. Sometimes patients could describe tinnitus and aural fullness at the unsuspected ear, and this may be a clue of a beginning of a bilateral involvement. In this case if surgery is considered to be offered, the procedures that preserve the hearing should be advised [26].

If vertical or perverted nystagmus is present, oculomotor test results are abnormal, or in order to suppress the nystagmus visual fixation fails, it indicates the central nervous system involvement. Intracranial lesion of posterior fossa lesions could mimic the symptoms of peripheral pathologies; in order to eliminate these conditions, gadolinium-enhanced MRI studies must be performed [65]. If the patients are at high risk of general anesthesia or surgery due to their general health problem, nonsurgical destructive treatment options should be considered.

If surgery is the decided treatment method, the next step is to decide on the procedure. The most important factor in decision process is hearing function of the patients and his perception of their hearing. If patient has a residual hearing and he/she finds it useful, then vestibular neurectomy, which is aimed to preserve hearing, should be advised. If no evidence of remaining hearing or patient cannot acknowledge the hearing on the affected side, labyrinthectomy, which destructs the remaining hearing function completely, should be advised.

French Otorhinolaryngology Head and Neck Surgery Society guideline of Meniere's disease management advises to start with less invasive and destructive procedures, such as ventilation tube placement and endolymphatic sac surgery. Especially in bilateral cases, clinician is advised to avoid from any destructive procedures. If these approaches are insufficient, destructive procedures should be considered according to the hearing function of the patient [4]. European position statement on Meniere's disease management advise the destructive procedures as the fifth and last line of treatment [5]. International Consensus (ICON) on treatment of Meniere's disease also keeps the destructive surgical options as the last resort [3].

Meniere's disease's progressive nature, the risk of bilateral involvement in any time of the life and possibility of spontaneous relief of vertigo in years always have to be kept in mind. Paparella recommended that treatment should be started with less invasive and destructive options; if the current treatment method seemed to fail, more invasive and destructive procedures should be considered [1].

3.3 Destructive procedures

3.3.1 Labyrinthectomy

If the affected side's hearing is not functional and the labyrinthine symptoms are recurrent, labyrinthectomy could be performed for any vestibular dysfunction.

If patients have profound hearing loss and have intractable vertigo or Tumarkin crisis and disease is unilateral, then labyrinthectomy should be considered [4]. It could be performed in a transcanal or transmastoid approach.

3.3.1.1 Transcanal labyrinthectomy

Tympanomeatal flap is elevated transcanally and middle ear is visualized. Stapes is removed from the oval window in order to access to the bony part of labyrinth. If visualization of the vestibule is needed, the bone from the promontory that lies below the oval window to round window could be removed. Saccule and utricule are identified and then removed. Access to the ampullae of the horizontal and superior semicircular canals is performed with a right angled instrument that is placed medial to the facial nerve and conducted with blind dissection. The bony part of the vestibule could be drilled to the round window to improve visualization and identification of the nerve that innervates the posterior semicircular canal, located to the posterior ampullae. Posterior semicircular canal nerve should be identified, and in order to not leave any residual PSCC function must be sectioned.

Some authors choose to pack the cavity with soluble packing materials that soaked with aminoglycoside, to prevent from its ototoxic effects and improve the surgery success.

3.3.1.2 Transmastoid labyrinthectomy

Transmastoid labyrinthectomy is a gold standard procedure of the vestibular function destruction. Mastoid cortex is presented in retroauricular approach. Cortical mastoidectomy is performed, and sinodural angle and middle fossa dura should be carefully dissected to have adequate visualization to facial nerve and access to the vestibule and posterior canal ampullae. The antrum is identified and the dome of horizontal semicircular canal is visualized at the depth. The largest bur that fits between middle fossa dura and horizontal semicircular canal should be chosen. The drilling must be deepened with solid angle between the three bony semicircular canals before any canal lumen is opened. Lumens of bony canals are opened from the internal surface of each canal toward the center of a deeper bony cup until the labyrinthine bone is removed completely.

Horizontal semicircular canal is an important landmark to identify the tympanic segment of the facial nerve so it usually opened first. The drill should never rise to a level that is lateral to the inferior lip of the bony cup to prevent facial nerve injury. After horizontal canal is opened, dissection is continued toward its nonampullated end until the superior canal is identified and opened. The posterior canal is followed to its ampulla end. At this site, bleeding from subarcuate artery is expected and should be controlled. Following the posterior canal, ampulla is opened which is adjacent to the horizontal canal ampulla.

Dissection stays inside the cup, and inner surface of the posterior canal must be followed to prevent the injury of the second genu of the facial nerve. By skeletonize the facial canal and removal of and bony structure to limit the visualization should be removed to protect the facial nerve. Drilling should be carried on to the parallel of the facial nerve canal. After the posterior canal ampulla is opened, the bone that connects the three ampullae is removed. All membranous labyrinth is carefully removed, and the thin bone at the lateral end of the internal acoustic canal should be preserved.

3.3.1.3 Complications

It is not a complication but an expected result, but the remaining hearing of the ipsilateral ear is lost with vestibular function. Nystagmus could persist for days, and most of the patients are able to move without any assistance in 2–3 days, but the complete vestibular compensation takes months. Disequilibrium could persist in some patients.

Possible complications are facial nerve injury, CSF leak, and chronic disequilibrium. The dura of the posterior cranial fossa or IAC must be preserved to prevent CSF leak or meningitis.

3.3.1.4 Results

Labyrinthectomy is the oldest procedure to treat Meniere's disease and gold standard. Wareing and O'Connor demonstrated that vertigo control rates of labyrinthectomy are 93–100%; however in longer follow-up 76% of the patients reported to have residual symptoms. Possible incomplete removal of the vestibular tissue might be the reason of recurrence in long term [66]. It is also reported that some patients have hard time of compensation, first 1 or 2 weeks of disequilibrium is expected but it could take months for fully compensation also inadequate removal of the vestibular tissue could cause these residual sysmptoms [67]. Vertigo control rates are superior compared to vestibular neurectomy or endolymphatic sac surgery [68].

3.3.2 Vestibular neurectomy

The aim of this procedure is to inhibit the inputs from peripheral vestibular system and prevent the cochlear nerve to protect remaining hearing. It has high vertigo control rates which vary from 80 to 95% but still not better than labyrinthectomy [26].

3.3.3 Translabyrinthine approach and transcochlear approach

For these approaches, common labyrinthectomy is performed. Then the dissection is carried on with intradural dissection of the vestibular nerve within IAC. The vestibular nerve is dissected to the medial of Scarpa's ganglion. After labyrinthectomy is performed in transmastoid approach, IAC dura is identified and opened. The division of vestibular nerve to superior and inferior is identified and sectioned.

Transcochlear approach begins with transcanal labyrinthectomy. Then the cochlea is opened and cochlear nerve is followed in IAC with vestibular nerve. This approach aims to decrease tinnitus. However these approaches contain high risk of CSF leak and meningitis, and desired results could be achieved with adequate transmastoid labyrinthectomy [69].

3.3.4 Middle fossa approach

House was the first surgeon to introduce middle fossa approach for vestibular neurectomy in 1961 [70]. Later it was improved by Fisch and Glasscock et al. in the 1970s [71–73].

It is a very refined surgical procedure, and vestibular nerve fibers are identified in the lateral part of IAC where the vestibular nerve separates from the cochlear nerve.

Temporal craniotomy that is centered to external auditory canal is performed. Dura is elevated from the temporal bone and the temporal lobe is retracted. Dura of IAC is skeletonized; in order to prevent further injury to the cochlea, superior semicircular canal, and facial nerve, dissection should be carried around IAC widely. First superior then inferior vestibular nerve are identified and sectioned. While sectioning of inferior vestibular nerve, labyrinthine artery must be preserved. This artery is located close to the inferior vestibular nerve at the distal part of IAC.

3.3.5 Retrolabyrinthine approach

Retrolabyrinthine approach for vestibular neurectomy was first described by Silverstein and Norrell [74, 75]. Retrolabyrinthine approach was developed in the 1980s, and it was reported to have lower facial nerve injury and hearing loss [75–77]. This procedure is also simpler than middle fossa approach. The eighth cranial nerve is only exposed between the brainstem and IAC; therefore it may be harder to identify auditory nerve than vestibular nerve specifically.

Dandy reported eighth cranial nerve section for vertigo treatment with suboccipital craniotomy in the 1930s, and long-term follow-up results were reported at 90% rate of complete vertigo control [78, 79]. This approach is named "retrosigmoid approach" nowadays.

The middle and posterior dura should be decompressed widely to get an ideal exposure, and retrosigmoid dura should be uncovered at least 1.5 cm posterior to the sigmoid sinus. This should allow enough extradural retraction. The bone that covers sigmoid sinus anteriorly is removed to the bony labyrinth's outline. Jugular bulb is the inferior limit of the dissection. Appropriate precautions should be taken to prevent the bone dust to enter the middle ear space.

The presigmoid dura and endolymphatic sac are incised parallel to sigmoid sinus to expose the posterior fossa dura. The cerebellum is retracted to visualize the cerebellopontine angle. Tentorium cerebelli and trigeminal nerve are identified superiorly, and the eighth cranial nerve is located inferiorly. This angle allows to visualize the posterior side of the petrous bone, so the internal acoustic canal is not visible. With minor retraction of the eighth cranial nerve, facial nerve could be visualized and advised to be controlled with electrostimulation. Vestibular fibers of the eighth nerve are located caudally (superiorly); this portion should be divided from the inferior portion of the nerve and separated with sharp dissection.

Musculus temporalis fascia is advised to be used for dural closure in order to prevent cerebrospinal fluid leak. The aditus ad antrum is blocked with fascia, and mastoidectomy defect is filled with harvested abdominal fat graft.

Retrosigmoid approach has some disadvantages such as the restricted recognition of vestibular and cochlear nerve, incomplete section of vestibular nerve, and possible damage to the cochlear nerve. However the hearing results of this approach were reported the same with other approaches. Postoperative headache is another significant trouble due to the intradural retraction of the cerebellum. Fukuhara et al. suggested the use of lumbar drainage for decompression of posterior fossa before the operation and reported that their operation time shortened, no CSF leakage occurred, and postoperative headache incidence is lowered [80].

Retrolabyrinthine-retrosigmoid combined approach was modified by Silverstein and his team in 1985. This modification allows effective access to cerebellopontine angle, and distinction of vestibular and cochlear nerve is clearer. Later they reported 85% of the patients had complete vertigo control, and the hearing preservation results were called "excellent." Only 20% of the patients had minor change at hearing, and only 4% of them experienced serious sensorineural hearing loss [81].

In order to identify cochlear and vestibular nerve clearer, some surgeons combine retrolabyrinthine approach with retrosigmoid approach. This procedure allows to remove the bone behind internal acoustic canal for better distinction of the nerve bundles [81, 82]. Retrolabyrinthine-retrosigmoid combined approach is still a gold standard in vestibular neurectomy procedure [83].

3.3.6 Infralabyrinthine approach

This technique is rarely used for vestibular neurectomy. The posterior semicircular canal is outlined, and the retrofacial air cells are tracted inferiorly. Internal acoustic canal is located inferiorly to the bony labyrinth.

Intradural dissection is limited to the internal acoustic canal's distal part, and vestibular nerve could be clearly identified while preserving the facial nerve. However poorly pneumatized temporal bones are hard to be dissected with this technique [84].

Intradural approaches for vestibular neurectomy could have serious complications such as stroke, subdural hematoma, and meningitis. Another life-changing complication is facial nerve paralysis, but rarely reported. Sensorineural hearing loss is another complication, reported in less than 10% of the cases [85].

3.3.6.1 Results

Most of the patients return to their daily lifestyle 2–4 months after the surgery.

Vertigo control rates of vestibular neurectomy is slightly worse than labyrinthectomy, reported 80–95% [86].

3.4 Comparison of surgical interventions

Surgery is the last resort for Meniere's disease. Most of the patients' symptoms could be taken under control with less invasive methods. If surgery is on the table, it is decided upon the patients hearing and general health performance. The ideal result of the surgery must control the vestibular symptoms completely while, if present, hearing should be preserved.

Endolymphatic sac decompression is frequently performed procedure if patient has remaining hearing function. Recent Cochrane review investigated the results of endolymphatic sac decompression with other procedures. Two randomized controlled studies were included. Bretlau et al. compared endolymphatic sac shunt to placebo procedure. Placebo procedure was simple mastoidectomy. The second study was by Thomsen et al.; they compared endolymphatic sac shunt to ventilation tube insertion. Vertigo control and hearing preservation were found the same at both studies. Bretlau reported the tinnitus was improved in both groups; however, Thomsen did not find any difference between the two groups. Both of the studies used different procedures as placebo and reported that 70% of their patients had been relieved of their symptoms regardless the procedure. However it is emphasized that the blinding of the studies were poor and methodic quality is low [22].

Moffat [87], Huang and Lin [88], Gibson [89], and Gianoli et al. [90] reported their 2-year results after endolymphatic sac surgery and reported that their vertigo control rates were 43.0, 84.4, 56.8, and 60.0%, while their hearing preservation with less than 10 dB loss or improvement 10 dB or more were reported 74.0, 83.4, 44.2, and 82.0%. However these studies were lack of comparison groups.

Kitahara et al. suggested that high dose of steroid administration during endolymphatic sac drainage to improve the effectiveness of the procedure. While the endolymphatic sac was opened in to mastoidectomy cavity, steroid was applied around the sac. All of their patients had intractable disease and are grouped blindly into two groups, while the group 1 was administered steroids during surgery and group 2 did not. Patients who had intractable disease but refused surgical intervention were used as control group, Group 3. Surgery group was reported to have better vertigo control rates than nonsurgery group after 7-year follow-up, while there was no significant difference between group 1 and group 2. Steroid-administered group 1's hearing function results were significantly better than group 2. Later they reported their findings in 2013 while including group 1 and nonsurgical group 3. Group 1 reported to have significantly better hearing and vertigo control rates [91].

Paparella and Fina investigated over 2000 patients who went through endolymphatic sac enhancement surgery. Seventy-five percent of the patients had complete relief from vertigo, and over 90% of them reported that their vertigo was improved. Only 5% of the patients had revision usually 3–4 years after the first procedure. They reported that hearing preservation was achieved over 98% of the patients, and 40% of the patients hearing were improved. Serious sensorineural hearing loss after endolymphatic sac procedure was reported only to be 2% [92].

Endolymphatic sac shunt and endolymphatic sac decompression are similar operations, and both of them have similar results like more than 70% of vertigo control [93]. Further investigations of shunt procedures according to their choice on silastic placement and direct shunting to mastoidectomy cavity. Patients' hearing functions were reported better when silastic tube had not been placed, but vertigo control rates were found similar (75.0–76.9%) [55, 91].

Endolymphatic sac surgery's safety in elder population is also investigated and established as safe. Sajjadi et al. presented their results in elder Meniere's disease patients aged 65 years and older. Seventy-seven percent of their patients reported to have complete relieve of vertigo in 2-year follow-up, and no significant complications, sequels, or deaths were reported. The most major complication that reported was cardiac arrhythmia which was recorded on 1.6% of the patients [94].

Vestibular neurectomy is another option while residual hearing presents. Vestibular neurectomy with middle cranial fossa approach had 90% or above at vertigo control while hearing preservation rates are reported to be 76–92% in 2-year follow-up. However the long-term results showed that vestibular neurectomy did not prevent the hearing loss progression, and 5–10 years after the procedure, nearly 50% of the patients had hearing loss [95, 96].

Quaranta et al. reported their findings on hearing preservation of patients who had vestibular neurectomy, another group who had endolymphatic sac surgery, and the group who refused to had any surgical interventions. Hearing preservation rates were 58.6% in vestibular neurectomy group, 58.8% in endolymphatic sac surgery group, and 50.0% of nonsurgical group in long-term follow-up, and no significant difference was found [97].

Recent review of Kitahara et al. reviewed the results of different surgical intervention results for intractable Meniere's disease in 5–10 years. They also included nonsurgical destructive treatment and intratympanic gentamicin administration's results. Over 90% of vestibular neurectomy cases, complete vertigo control achieved while intratympanic gentamicin control rates were over 80%, endolymphatic sac surgery control rates were 70–80% and nonsurgical group vertigo control rates were 25–70%. They also evaluated the hearing function preservation (10 dB or higher) [93]. Their results were summarized in **Table 3**.

While vestibular neurectomy is superior to control vertigo attacks, endolymphatic sac surgery has better hearing preservation rates.

Labyrinthectomy is still the gold standard to control peripheral vertigo. However it is a highly destructive procedure. It destroys peripheral vestibular organ as well as the remaining hearing function. It is advised for patients who had total

	Complete vertigo control (%)	Hearing preservation >10 dB (%)
Vestibular neurectomy	>90	50–60
Intratympanic gentamicin	>80	50–60
Endolymphatic sac surgery	70–80	60–80
Nonsurgical	25–70	25–50

Table 3.
Results of interventions to intractable Meniere's disease in 5–10 years.

hearing loss at the affected ear. Selective vestibular neurectomy has advantages on this subject. Vestibular neurectomy interrupts the vestibular input while preserving the hearing functions. Both of these procedures have very successful vertigo control rates (98.8% for labyrinthectomy and 97.8% for vestibular neurectomy) [98–101].

De la Cruz et al. conducted a study to investigate the efficacy of surgical treatment modalities. They evaluated 3637 procedures that were performed on 30-year period, such as endolymphatic sac shunt, vestibular nerve section (translabyrinthine, retrolabyrinthine, retrosigmoid, and middle fossa approaches), and labyrinthectomy. They assessed the outcomes of these procedures with a questionnaire. Vertigo characteristics were reported to be improved at each group; endolymphatic sac shunt and vestibular neurectomy groups also had stated that their balance was improved. Some of the patients who had labyrinthectomy reported that their imbalance worsened after surgery. All groups reported that they still have some balance problems, while endolymphatic sac shunt group had less problems, and labyrinthectomy group's balance problems were worse than the other groups [102]. Glasscock et al. [103], Schuknecht [104], and Kemink et al. [105] also reported similar results.

It is reported that some patients' vertigo attacks were recurred after vestibular neurectomy. Incomplete nerve section, neuroma formation, inadequate compensation, vestibular disorder at the contralateral side, and unwanted nerve regeneration were suggested as an explanation for these cases [106].

Vestibular neurectomy with translabyrinthine approach and labyrinthectomy results is expected to be similar. De la Cruz et al. also compared these sub-groups with each other and found that over 80% of each group had complete control of vertigo; however labyrinthectomy groups stated that their current imbalance is more severe than the translabyrinthine vestibular neurectomy group [102]; similar results were reported by different authors [103–105].

Surgical outcomes are also related with preoperative factors. Teufert et al. designed a study to assess the prognostic factors that could affect surgical outcomes. They assessed patients with the AAO-HNS vertigo score and class, number of vertigo attacks per month, current and change in AAO-HNS disability rating, and vertigo and imbalance severity ratings and imbalance frequency. AAO-HNS disability rating, imbalance frequency and duration of symptoms were found related to outcome. Higher disability ratings and more frequent imbalance are related with poorer outcomes. Longer the symptoms had been presented, related with better outcome. The characteristic of the vertigo was not associated with outcome. Also patients who had contralateral tinnitus had worse outcome. If the first symptom was vertigo, tinnitus was present at contralateral side, and poor visual function is also found to be related with poor outcome [107].

In conclusion, there are many surgical procedures present nowadays, and each one of them has advantages as well as disadvantages. Some of the results were predictable, like hearing loss after labyrinthectomy. However surgeon must assess the patient thoroughly and choose the most appropriate procedure for him/her.

The outcome has a very close relationship with patients' psychological state. Patients who did not have any psychological problems were reported to have better outcomes from treatment (surgical or nonsurgical). Surgical procedures found to be more effective than nonsurgical treatment at the patients with psychological problems [62].

4. Vestibular compensation after the surgery

It could take months to compensate the loss of unilateral vestibular input. Thirty percent of the patients were reported to have disequilibrium after the vestibular surgery. Pereira and Kerr demonstrated that most patients after labyrinthectomy reported that their vertigo had been relieved completely, but only 50% of them were able to return to their routine lifestyles [108]. Vertigo control is the first goal of the surgery, but compensation after surgery should not be underestimated.

The recovery after vestibular neurectomy is reported longer than labyrinthectomy and usually more incomplete; it is reported that postoperative ataxia incidence of vestibular neurectomy is 11%, but labyrinthectomy rates are reported 2% [109].

Vestibular rehabilitation is mandatory for all patients before and after the surgery. The rehabilitation program should be customized for each patient. Patients who had additional sensory deficit, visual problems, or neurologic conditions are candidates for delayed recovery. Psychological factors also play an important role in recovery phase.

Labyrinthectomy failures could occur if the diagnosis had been wrong or the neuroepithelium removal had been performed incompletely. Vestibular compensation of these patients was inadequate. Late failures of this procedure could be a result of central decompensation, but it responds to vestibular rehabilitation [110].

Vestibular neurectomy failures are usually associated with incomplete section of the vestibular nerve fibers. If the condition worsens, revision surgery should be considered.

Vestibular rehabilitation has a very important role after vestibular neurectomy and labyrinthectomy. Both procedures cause a complete loss of unilateral vestibular function. Vestibular rehabilitation is accepted as the best way to improve imbalance problems and regenerate patients' daily functions. The rehabilitation program must be customized. The somatosensory system is the first one to adapt, disequilibrium reduces within 3 weeks, and postural stability prevails months after [111].

Author details

Yetkin Zeki Yilmaz[1*], Begum Bahar Yilmaz[1] and Mehmet Yilmaz[2]

1 ENT, Cerrahpasa Medical Faculty, Istanbul University, Istanbul, Turkey

2 Yunus Emre Clinic, Turkey

*Address all correspondence to: dr_yzy@hotmail.com

References

[1] Sajjadi H, Paparella MM. Meniere's disease. Lancet. 2008. DOI: 10.1016/S0140-6736(08)61161-7

[2] Arenberg I. Proposition for endolymphatic sac and duct surgery. In: Arenberg I, Graham MD, editors. Treatment Options for Meniere's Disease. Singular Publishing; 1998. pp. 19-23

[3] Nevoux J, Barbara M, Dornhoffer J, Gibson W, Kitahara T, Darrouzet V. International consensus (ICON) on treatment of Ménière's disease. European Annals of Otorhinolaryngology, Head and Neck Diseases. 2018. DOI: 10.1016/j.anorl.2017.12.006

[4] Nevoux J, Franco-Vidal V, Bouccara D, et al. Diagnostic and therapeutic strategy in Menière's disease. Guidelines of the French Otorhinolaryngology-Head and Neck Surgery Society (SFORL). European Annals of Otorhinolaryngology, Head and Neck Diseases. 2017. DOI: 10.1016/j.anorl.2016.12.003

[5] Magnan J, Ozgirgin ON, Trabalzini F, et al. European position statement on diagnosis, and treatment of Meniere's disease. The Journal of International Advanced Otology. 2018;**14**(2):317-321. DOI: 10.5152/iao.2018.140818

[6] Nakashima T, Naganawa S, Sugiura M, et al. Visualization of endolymphatic hydrops in patients with Meniere's disease. The Laryngoscope. 2007;**117**(3):415-420. DOI: 10.1097/MLG.0b013e31802c300c

[7] Naganawa S, Yamazaki M, Kawai H, Bokura K, Sone M, Nakashima T. Visualization of endolymphatic hydrops in Ménière's disease with single-dose intravenous gadolinium-based contrast media using heavily T2-weighted 3D-FLAIR. Magnetic Resonance in Medical Sciences. 2010. DOI: 10.2463/mrms.9.237

[8] Naganawa S, Nakashima T. Visualization of endolymphatic hydrops with MR imaging in patients with Ménière's disease and related pathologies: Current status of its methods and clinical significance. Japanese Journal of Radiology. 2014. DOI: 10.1007/s11604-014-0290-4

[9] De Sousa LCA, De Toledo Piza MR, Da Costa SS. Diagnosis of Meniere's disease: Routine and extended tests. Otolaryngologic Clinics of North America. 2002. DOI: 10.1016/S0030-6665(02)00029-4

[10] Paparella MM. Methods of diagnosis and treatment of Meniere's disease. Acta Oto-Laryngologica. 1991. DOI: 10.3109/00016489109128050

[11] Paparella MM, Mcdermott JC, Sousa LCA. Meniere's disease and the peak audiogram. Archives of Otolaryngology. 1982. DOI: 10.1001/archotol.1982.00790570021005

[12] Dobie RA, Snyder JM, Donaldson JA. Electronystagmographic and audiologic findings in patients with Meniere's disease. Acta Oto-Laryngologica. 1982. DOI: 10.3109/00016488209128885

[13] Young Y-H, Huang T-W, Cheng P-W. Vestibular evoked myogenic potentials in delayed endolymphatic hydrops. The Laryngoscope. 2002; **112**(9):1623-1626. DOI: 10.1097/00005537-200209000-00018

[14] Nedzelski JM, Schessel DA, Bryce GE, Pfleiderer AG. Chemical labyrinthectomy: Local application of gentamicin for the treatment of unilateral Menière's disease. The American Journal of Otology. 1992

[15] Doyle KJ, Bauch C, Battista R, et al. Intratympanic steroid treatment: A review. Otology & Neurotology. 2004. DOI: 10.1097/00129492-200411000-00031

[16] Claes J, Van De Heyning PH. A review of medical treatment for Ménière's disease. Acta Oto-Laryngologica. 2000. DOI: 10.1080/000164800750044461

[17] Santos PM, Hall RA, Snyder JM, Hughes LF, Dobie RA. Diuretic and diet effect on Meniere's disease evaluated by the 1985 committee on hearing and equilibrium guidelines. Otolaryngology - Head and Neck Surgery. 1993. DOI: 10.1177/019459989310900408

[18] Konrad HR. Intractable vertigo—When not to operate. Otolaryngology - Head and Neck Surgery. 1986. DOI: 10.1177/019459988609500411

[19] Monsell EM, Brackmann DE, Linthicum FH. Why do vestibular destructive procedures sometimes fail? Otolaryngology - Head and Neck Surgery. 1988. DOI: 10.1177/019459988809900505

[20] Wiet RJ, Kazan R, Shambaugh GEJ. An holistic approach to Meniere's disease. Medical and surgical management. The Laryngoscope. 1981

[21] Charpiot A, Rohmer D, Gentine A. Lateral semicircular canal plugging in severe Ménière's disease: A clinical prospective study about 28 patients. Otology & Neurotology. 2010. DOI: 10.1097/MAO.0b013e3181ca85a2

[22] Pullens B, Hp V, Pp VB. Surgery for Ménière's disease (review). 2013;(2)

[23] Schuknecht HF, Bartley M. Cochlear endolymphatic shunt for Meniere's disease. The American Journal of Otology. 1985

[24] Schuknecht HF. Cochleosacculotomy for Meniere's disease: Internal endolymphatic shunt. Operative Techniques in Otolaryngology-Head and Neck Surgery. 1991. DOI: 10.1016/S1043-1810(10)80227-1

[25] Kinney WC, Nalepa N, Hughes GB, Kinney SE. Cochleosacculotomy for the treatment of Meniere's disease in the elderly patient. The Laryngoscope. 1995. DOI: 10.1288/00005537-199509000-00012

[26] Telian SA, Basura GJ. Surgery for vestibular disorders. In: Flint PW, Haughey BH, Lund VJ, et al., editors. Cummings Otolaryngology: Head and Neck Surgery. 6th ed. Saunders: Canada; 2015. pp. 2581-2593

[27] Yamakawa K. Über die pathologische Veränderung bei einem Meniere-Kranken. Journal of Otolaryngology. 1938;**44**:2310-2312

[28] Hallpike CS, Cairns H. Observations on the pathology of Ménière's syndrome. Proceedings of the Royal Society of Medicine. 1938. DOI: 10.1017/S0022215100003947

[29] Committee on Hearing and Equilibrium guidelines for the diagnosis and evaluation of therapy in Meniere's disease. Otolaryngology - Head and Neck Surgery. 1995. DOI: 10.1016/S0194-5998(95)70102-8

[30] Kaufman AI. Viral theory for Meniere's disease and endolymphatic hydrops: Overview and new therapeutic options for viral labyrinthitis. Annals of the New York Academy of Sciences. 1997. DOI: 10.1111/j.1749-6632.1997.tb51901.x

[31] Kimura RS, Schuknecht HF, Ota CY, Jones DD. Obliteration of the ductus reuniens. Acta Oto-Laryngologica. 1980. DOI: 10.3109/00016488009127141

[32] Paparella MM. Pathogenesis and pathophysiology of Meniere's disease. Acta Oto-Laryngologica. 1991. DOI: 10.3109/00016489109128041

[33] Zechner G, Altmann F. Histological studies on the human endolymphatic duct and sac. Practica oto-Rhino-Laryngologica. 1969;**31**:65-83

[34] Sando I, Ikeda M. The vestibular aqueduct in patients with Meniere's disease: A temporal bone histopathological investigation. Acta Oto-Laryngologica. 1984. DOI: 10.3109/00016488409132934

[35] Ikeda M, Sando I. Endolymphatic duct and sac in patients with Meniere's disease: A temporal bone histopathological study. The Annals of Otology, Rhinology, and Laryngology. 1984. DOI: 10.1177/000348948409300603

[36] Paparella MM, Sajjadi H. Endolymphatic sac revision for recurrent Meniere's disease. The American Journal of Otology. 1988

[37] Paparella M, Sajjadi H. Endolymphatic sac procedures. In: Brackmann DE, Shelton C, Arriaga M, editors. Otologic Surgery. Philadelphia: WB Saunders; 2001. pp. 371-384

[38] Arts HA, Kileny PR, Telian SA. Diagnostic testing for endolymphatic hydrops. Otolaryngologic Clinics of North America. 1997

[39] Portmann G. Surgical treatment of vertigo by opening of the saccus endolymphaticus. Archives of Otolaryngology. 1969. DOI: 10.1001/archotol.1969.00770020811005

[40] House W. Subarachnoid shunt for drainage of endolymphatic hydrops. The Laryngoscope. 1962;**72**:713-729

[41] Paparella MM, And CSK, Shea DA. Sac decompression for refractory luetic vertigo. Acta Oto-Laryngologica. 1980. DOI: 10.3109/00016488009127172

[42] Graham MD, Kemink JL. Surgical management of Meniere's disease with endolymphatic sac decompression by wide bony decompression of the posterior fossa dura: Technique and results. The Laryngoscope. 1984

[43] Ostrowski VB, Kartush JM. Endolymphatic sac-vein decompression for intractable Meniere's disease: Long term treatment results. Otolaryngology - Head and Neck Surgery. 2003. DOI: 10.1016/S0194-5998(03)00084-6

[44] Chung JW, Fayad J, Linthicum F, Ishiyama A, Merchant SN. Histopathology after endolymphatic sac surgery for Ménière's syndrome. Otology & Neurotology. 2011. DOI: 10.1097/MAO.0b013e31821553ce

[45] Linthicum FH, Santos F. Endolymphatic sac amputation without hydrops. Otology & Neurotology. 2011. DOI: 10.1097/MAO.0b013e3181db733e

[46] Saliba I, Gabra N, Alzahrani M, Berbiche D. Endolymphatic duct blockage: A randomized controlled trial of a novel surgical technique for Ménière's disease treatment. Otolaryngology - Head and Neck Surgery. 2015. DOI: 10.1177/0194599814555840

[47] Sennaroglu L, Sennaroglu G, Gursel B, Dini FM. Intratympanic dexamethasone, intratympanic gentamicia and endolymphatic sac surgery for intractable vertigo in Meniere's disease. Otolaryngology - Head and Neck Surgery. 2001. DOI: 10.1067/mhn.2001.119485

[48] Silverstein H, Smouha E, Jones R. Natural history vs. surgery for Meniere's disease. Otolaryngology - Head and Neck Surgery. 1989. DOI: 10.1177/019459988910000102

[49] Jackson CG, Dickins JR, McMenomey SO, et al. Endolymphatic system shunting: A long-term profile of the Denver inner ear shunt. The American Journal of Otology. 1996

[50] Smith DR, Pyle GM. Outcome-based assessment of endolymphatic sac surgery for Meniere's disease. The Laryngoscope. 1997. DOI: 10.1097/00005537-199709000-00010

[51] Pensak ML, Friedman RA. The role of endolymphatic mastoid shunt surgery in the managed care era. The American Journal of Otology. 1998

[52] Huang TS, Lin CC, Chang YL. Endolymphatic sac surgery for Meniere's disease: A cumulative study of twelve years' experience. Acta Oto-Laryngologica. 1991. DOI: 10.3109/00016489109128054

[53] Welling DB, Nagaraja HN. Endolymphatic mastoid shunt: A reevaluation of efficacy. Otolaryngology - Head and Neck Surgery. 2000. DOI: 10.1067/mhn.2000.101575

[54] Huang TS. Endolymphatic sac surgery for Meniere's disease: Experience with over 3000 cases. Otolaryngologic Clinics of North America. 2002. DOI: 10.1016/S0030-6665(02)00027-0

[55] Kitahara T, Fukushima M, Uno A, et al. Long-term results of endolymphatic sac drainage with local steroids for intractable Meniere's disease. Auris, Nasus, Larynx. 2013. DOI: 10.1016/j.anl.2012.11.008

[56] Pullens B, Verschuur HP, Van Benthem PP. Surgery for Ménière's disease. Cochrane Database of Systematic Reviews 2013. doi:10.1002/14651858.CD005395.pub3

[57] Sood AJ, Lambert PR, Nguyen SA, Meyer TA. Endolymphatic sac surgery for ménière's disease: A systematic review and meta-analysis. Otology & Neurotology. 2014;**35**(6):1033-1045. DOI: 10.1097/MAO.0000000000000324

[58] Vereeck L, Wuyts FL, Truijen S, De Valck C, Van de Heyning PH. The effect of early customized vestibular rehabilitation on balance after acoustic neuroma resection. Clinical Rehabilitation. 2008. DOI: 10.1177/0269215508089066

[59] Enticott JC, O'Leary SJ, Briggs RJS. Effects of vestibulo-ocular reflex exercises on vestibular compensation after vestibular schwannoma surgery. Otology & Neurotology. 2005. DOI: 10.1097/00129492-200503000-00024

[60] Tjernström F, Fransson PA, Kahlon B, et al. Vestibular PREHAB and gentamicin before schwannoma surgery may improve long-term postural function. Journal of Neurology, Neurosurgery, and Psychiatry. 2009. DOI: 10.1136/jnnp.2008.170878

[61] Gottshall KR, Topp SG, Hoffer ME. Early vestibular physical therapy rehabilitation for Meniere's disease. Otolaryngologic Clinics of North America. 2010;**43**(5):1113-1119. DOI: 10.1016/j.otc.2010.05.006

[62] Yokota Y, Kitahara T, Sakagami M, et al. Surgical results and psychological status in patients with intractable Ménière's disease. Auris, Nasus, Larynx. 2016;**43**(3):287-291. DOI: 10.1016/j.anl.2015.10.007

[63] Telian SASNT. Update on vestibular rehabilitation therapy. Otolaryngologic Clinics of North America. 1996

[64] Shone G, Kemink JL, Telian SA, Shone GR. Prognostic significance of hearing loss as a lateralizing indicator in the surgical treatment of vertigo. The Journal of Laryngology and Otology. 1991. DOI: 10.1017/S0022215100116834

[65] Disher M, Telian S, Kemink JL. Evaluation of acute vertigo: Unusual lesions imitating vestibular neuritis. The American Journal of Otology. 1991; **12**(3):227-231

[66] Wareing MJ, O'Connor AF. The role of labyrinthectomy and cochlear implantation in Meniere's disease. Ear, Nose, & Throat Journal. 1997

[67] Alarcón AV, Hidalgo LOV, Arévalo RJ, Diaz MP. Labyrinthectomy and vestibular neurectomy for intractable vertiginous symptoms. International Archives of Otorhinolaryngology. 2017. DOI: 10.1055/s-0037-1599242

[68] Kartush J. Endolymphatic sac surgery. In: Arriaga M, editor. Essentials of Neurotology. London: Thieme; 2002

[69] Langman AW, Lindeman RC. Surgery for vertigo in the nonserviceable hearing ear: Transmastoid labyrinthectomy or translabyrinthine vestibular nerve section. The Laryngoscope. 1993. DOI: 10.1288/00005537-199312000-00001

[70] House W. Surgical exposure of the internal auditory canal and its contents through the middle cranial fossa. The Laryngoscope. 1961;**71**:1363

[71] Fisch U. Vestibular and cochlear neurectomy. Transactions of the American Academy of Ophthalmology and Otolaryngology. 1974;**78**(4):252-255

[72] Glasscock M 3rd. Vestibular nerve section. Middle fossa and translabyrinthine. Archives of Otolaryngology. 1973;**97**(2):112-114

[73] Glasscock ME, Kveton JF, Christiansen SG. Middle fossa vestibular neurectomy: An update. Otolaryngology - Head and Neck Surgery. 1984. DOI: 10.1177/019459988409200215

[74] Silverstein H, Norrell H. Retrolabyrinthine surgery: A direct approach to the cerebellopontine angle. In: Silverstein H, Norrell H, editors. Neurological Surgery of the Ear. Birmingham, AL: Aesculapius; 1979. pp. 318-322

[75] Silverstein H, Norrell H. Retrolabyrinthine surgery: A direct approach to the cerebellopontine angle. Otolaryngology - Head and Neck Surgery. 1980. DOI: 10.1177/019459988008800425

[76] House JW, Hitselberger WE, Mcelveen J, Brackmann DE. Retrolabyrinthine section of the vestibular nerve. Otolaryngology - Head and Neck Surgery. 1984. DOI: 10.1177/019459988409200214

[77] Kemink JL, Hoff JT. Retrolabyrinthine vestibular nerve section: Analysis of results. The Laryngoscope. 1986

[78] Dandy WE. Benign, encapsulated tumors in the lateral ventricles of the brain. The Journal of Nervous and Mental Disease. 2006. DOI: 10.1097/00005053-193510000-00042

[79] Green R. Surgical treatment of vertigo with follow up on Walter Dandy's cases. In: Proceedings of the Congress of Neurological Surgeons. Baltimore: Williams and Williams; 1958. p. 141

[80] Fukuhara T, Silverman DA, Hughes GB, et al. Vestibular nerve sectioning for intractable vertigo: Efficacy of simplified retrosigmoid approach. Otology & Neurotology. 2002. DOI: 10.1097/00129492-200201000-00016

[81] Silverstein H, Norrell H, Smouha EE. Retrosigmoid-internal auditory canal approach vs. retrolabyrinthine approach for vestibular neurectomy. Otolaryngology - Head and

Neck Surgery. 1987. DOI: 10.1177/019459988709700309

[82] McKenna MJ, Nadol JB Jr, Ojemann RG, Halpin C. Vestibular neurectomy: Retrosigmoid-intracanalicular versus retrolabyrinthine approach. The American Journal of Otology. 1996

[83] Silverstein H, Norrell H, Smouha E, Jones R. Combined retrolab-retrosigmoid vestibular neurectomy. An evolution in approach. The American Journal of Otology. 1989

[84] Vernick DM. Infralabyrinthine approach to the internal auditory canal. Otolaryngology - Head and Neck Surgery. 1990. DOI: 10.1177/019459989010200401

[85] Moody-Antonio S, House JW. Hearing outcome after concurrent endolymphatic shunt and vestibular nerve section. Otology & Neurotology. 2003. DOI: 10.1097/00129492-200305000-00016

[86] Green JD, Shelton C, Brackmann DE. Middle fossa vestibular neurectomy in retrolabyrinthine neurectomy failures. Archives of Otolaryngology - Head and Neck Surgery. 1992. DOI: 10.1001/archotol.1992.01880100048012

[87] Moffat DA. Endolymphatic sac surgery: Analysis of 100 operations. Clinical Otolaryngology and Allied Sciences. 1994. DOI: 10.1111/j.1365-2273.1994.tb01228.x

[88] Huang TS, Lin CC. Endolymphatic sac ballooning surgery for Meniere's disease. The Annals of Otology, Rhinology, and Laryngology. 1994. DOI: 10.1177/000348949410300509

[89] Gibson WPR. The effect of surgical removal of the extraosseous portion of the endolymphatic sac in patients suffering from Meniere's disease. The Journal of Laryngology and Otology. 1996. DOI: 10.1017/S0022215100135637

[90] Gianou GJ, Larouere MJ, Kartush JM, Wayman J. Sac-vein decompression for intractable Meniere's disease: Two-year treatment results. Otolaryngology - Head and Neck Surgery. 1998. DOI: 10.1016/S0194-5998(98)70370-5

[91] Kitahara T, Kubo T, Okumura SI, Kitahara M. Effects of endolymphatic sac drainage with steroids for intractable Ménière's disease: A long-term follow-up and randomized controlled study. The Laryngoscope. 2008. DOI: 10.1097/MLG.0b013e3181651c4a

[92] Paparella M. Revision of endolymphatic sac surgery for recurrent Meniere's disease. Otolaryngologic Clinics of North America. 2002;**35**(3):607-619. DOI: 10.1016/S0030-6665(02)00032-4

[93] Kitahara T. Evidence of surgical treatments for intractable Meniere's disease. Auris, Nasus, Larynx. 2018;**45**(3):393-398. DOI: 10.1016/j.anl.2017.07.016

[94] Sajjadi H, Paparella MM, Williams T. Endolymphatic sac enhancement surgery in elderly patients with Meniere's disease. Ear, Nose, & Throat Journal. 1998

[95] Silverstein H, Rosenberg S, Arruda J, Isaacson JE. Surgical ablation of the vestibular system in the treatment of Meniere's disease. Otolaryngologic Clinics of North America. 1997

[96] Tewary AK, Riley N, Kerr AG. Long-term results of vestibular nerve section. The Journal of Laryngology and Otology. 1998. DOI: 10.1017/S0022215100142719

[97] Quaranta A, Onofri M, Sallustio V, Iurato S. Comparison of long-term

hearing results after vestibular neurectomy, endolymphatic mastoid shunt, and medical therapy. The American Journal of Otology. 1997

[98] Fisch U. Middle fossa vestibular neurectomy. In: Silverstein H, Norrell H, editors. Neurological Surgery of the Ear. Aesculapius; 1977

[99] Hammerschlag PE, Schuknecht HF. Transcanal labyrinthectomy for intractable vertigo. Archives of Otolaryngology. 1981. DOI: 10.1001/archotol.1981.00790390018006

[100] Levine SC, Glasscock M, McKennan KX. Long-term results of labyrinthectomy. The Laryngoscope. 2006. DOI: 10.1288/00005537-199002000-00003

[101] Iurato S, Onofri M. A five to thirteen year follow-up of thirty-one consecutive cases of vestibular neurectomy for Meniere's disease. In: Nadol JBJ, editor. Second International Symposium on Meniere's Disease. Cambridge; 1988. pp. 563-566

[102] De la Cruz A, Teufert KB, Berliner KI. Surgical treatment for vertigo: Patient survey of vertigo, imbalance, and time course for recovery. Otolaryngology - Head and Neck Surgery. 2006. DOI: 10.1016/j.otohns.2006.05.011

[103] Glasscock ME, Davis WE, Hughes GB, Jackson CG. Labyrinthectomy versus middle fossa vestibular nerve section in Menière's disease; a critical evaluation of relief of vertigo. The Annals of Otology, Rhinology, and Laryngology. 1980. DOI: 10.1177/000348948008900405

[104] Schuknecht HF. Behavior of the vestibular nerve following labyrinthectomy. The Annals of Otology, Rhinology, and Laryngology. 1982

[105] Kemink JL, Telian SA, Graham MD, Joynt L. Transmastoid labyrinthectomy: Reliable surgical management of vertigo. Otolaryngology - Head and Neck Surgery. 1989. DOI: 10.1177/019459988910100102

[106] Thedinger BS, Thedinger BA. Analysis of patients with persistent dizziness after vestibular nerve section. Ear, Nose, & Throat Journal. 1998

[107] Teufert KB, Berliner KI, De La Cruz A. Persistent dizziness after surgical treatment of vertigo: An exploratory study of prognostic factors. Otology & Neurotology. 2007. DOI: 10.1097/MAO.0b013e318157fdd0

[108] Pereira KD, Kerr AG. Disabililty after labyrinthectomy. The Journal of Laryngology and Otology. 2007. DOI: 10.1017/s0022215100133237

[109] Gacek RR, Gacek MR. Comparison of labyrinthectomy and vestibular neurectomy in the control of vertigo. The Laryngoscope. 1996;**106**(2): 225-230. DOI: 10.1097/00005537-199602000-00023

[110] Katsarkas A, Segal BN. Unilateral loss of peripheral vestibular function in patients: Degree of compensation and factors causing decompensation. Otolaryngology - Head and Neck Surgery. 1988. DOI: 10.1177/019459988809800108

[111] Magnusson M, Kahlon B, Karlberg M, Lindberg S, Siesjö P, Tjernström F. Vestibular "pREHAB.". Annals of the New York Academy of Sciences. 2009. DOI: 10.1111/j.1749-6632.2009.03778.x